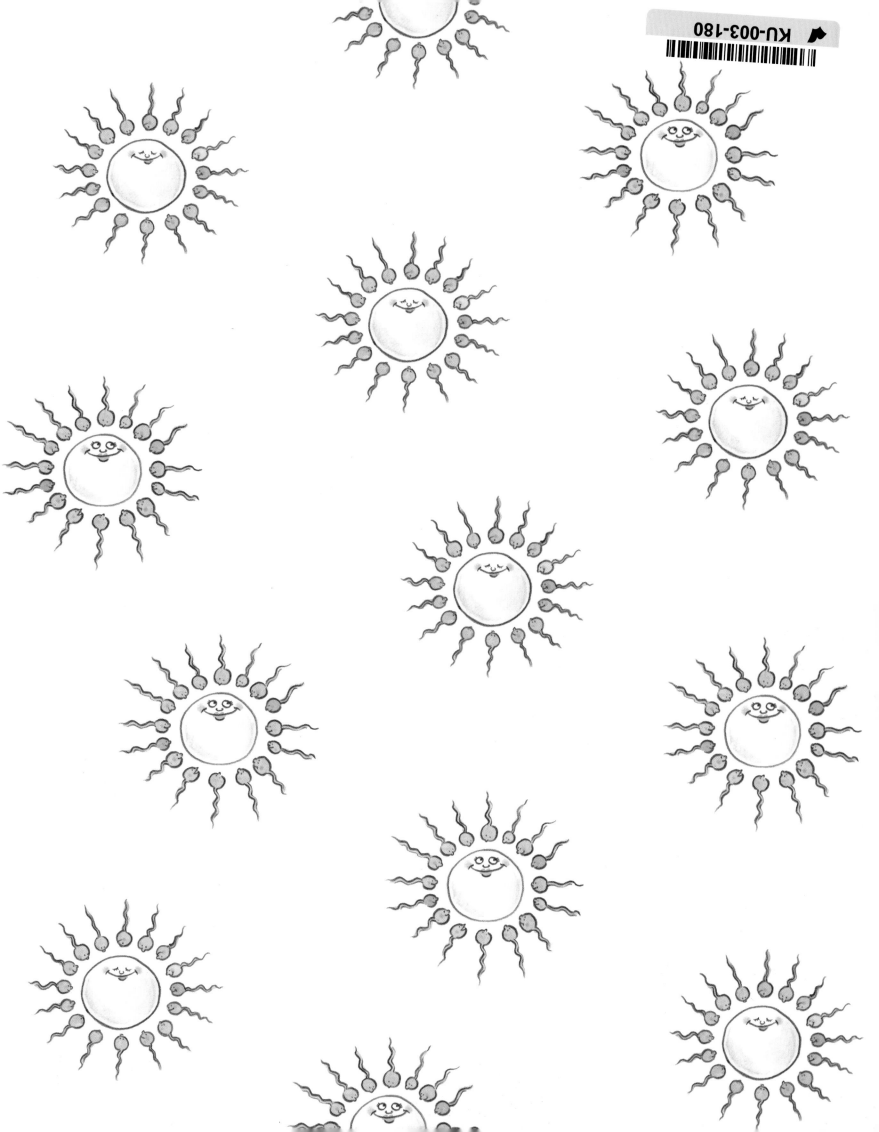

For Elaine Markson

A NOTE FROM THE AUTHOR AND THE ILLUSTRATOR
While writing the words and making the drawings for this book, we talked with children and
parents to find out what they wanted to know. We also talked with teachers, librarians,
scientists, doctors, nurses and clergy members. We asked all of them questions — over and over again.
We did all this because we wanted to make sure that the information, the words and the
drawings in this book would be useful, correct and as up-to-date as possible.

One of the most exciting and interesting things about making this book has been all that we
have learned from the people who talked with us and taught us. We also learned that science can change,
that not all scientists agree, that there are not always answers to every question and that
there can be more than one answer to a question.

At this time, the information in this book is as up-to-date as possible.
But if you have new questions, or more questions, or any questions at all, it can be
very helpful to talk with your parent, doctor, nurse, health professional, teacher, librarian,
school counsellor or clergy member.

Robie H. Harris and Michael Emberley
May 2002

The designs of the BIRD and the BEE are trademarks of BIRD Productions, Inc., and BEE Productions, Inc.
LET'S TALK ABOUT WHERE BABIES COME FROM is an IT'S PERFECTLY NORMAL book, which is a trademark of
BEE Productions, Inc., and BIRD Productions, Inc.

IT'S PERFECTLY NORMAL is the trademark of BEE Productions, Inc., and BIRD Productions, Inc.

Text ©1999 BEE Productions, Inc.
Illustrations ©1999 BIRD Productions, Inc.

First published 1999 by Walker Books Ltd
87 Vauxhall Walk, London SE11 5HJ

This edition published 2002

2 4 6 8 10 9 7 5 3 1

This book has been typeset in Providence Sans and Bookman

Printed in Hong Kong

British Library Cataloguing in Publication Data:
a catalogue record for this book is
available from the British Library

ISBN 0-7445-7756-X

LET'S TALK ABOUT
WHERE BABIES
COME FROM

A Book about Eggs, Sperm, Birth, Babies and Families

So what sex is it?

Boy?

A girl?

It's a boy!

Girl?

?!

Robie H. Harris

illustrated by
Michael Emberley

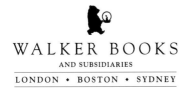

WALKER BOOKS
AND SUBSIDIARIES
LONDON • BOSTON • SYDNEY

CONTENTS

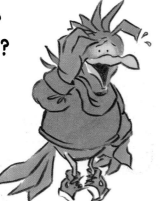

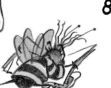

MEET THE BIRD AND THE BEE
Do You Know What I Read?

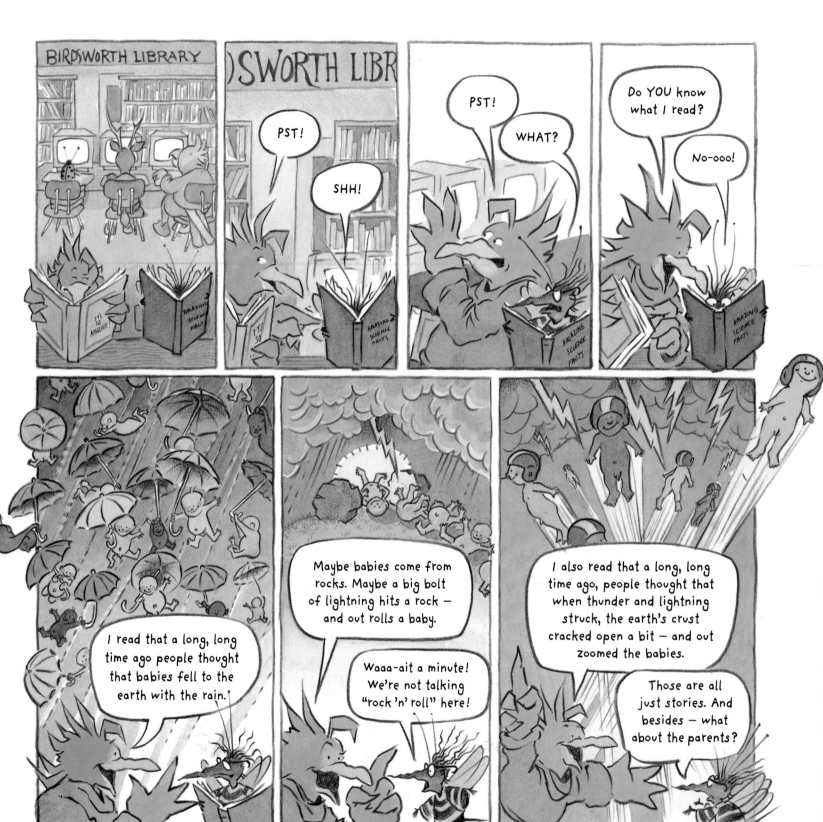

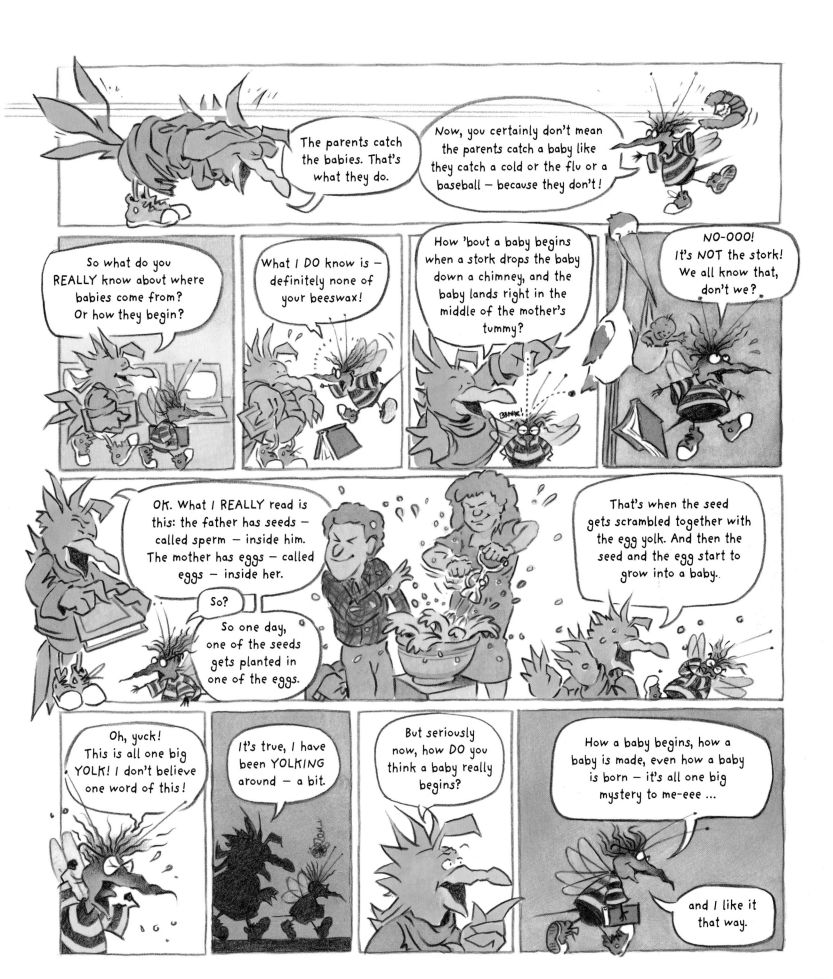

① CURIOUS? EMBARRASSED? CONFUSED?

So How Do Babies Really Begin?

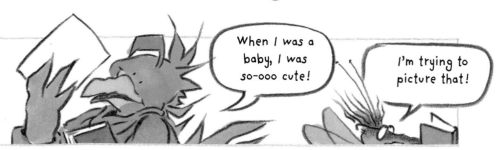

Have you ever looked at pictures of yourself as a baby?

Have you ever wondered where babies come from, or how babies are made, or where you came from, or how you really began?

Everyone – grandparents, parents, sisters, brothers, cousins, aunts, uncles, friends, and even teachers, firefighters, librarians, gymnasts, astronauts, dentists, scientists, cooks, nurses, shopkeepers, doctors, bus drivers, pilots, police officers, hockey players, mayors and rock stars – every person in the whole wide world was a baby once. The arrival of a new baby is so amazing! Most children – but not all – are curious about how such an amazing and wonderful thing could possibly happen.

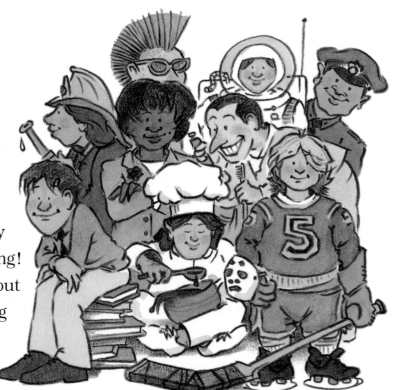

You may think that by now you already know – or that you should know – exactly how a baby is made. But even if your mum or dad has talked to you about this, or even if you and your friends have talked about it, it's still perfectly normal to have questions about where babies come from. Talking with a parent, a doctor, a nurse or a teacher is a good way to find out answers to your questions.

I'm so glad it's normal to have questions about THAT!

I have questions about dinosaurs, about outer space, but NOT about babies!

Sometimes you may feel very private about your questions and thoughts and feelings about how babies begin. Or it may feel embarrassing or hard to ask questions about making babies. Feeling curious about this, or embarrassed, or private, or even confused, is perfectly normal. And having lots of questions about where babies come from is also perfectly normal.

I can't WAIT to find out more about this!

I CAN wait.

Since the beginning of time, people young and old have tried to work out where babies come from and how a baby is made. But how a baby is made is not a simple thing. That's why learning about it can be interesting and even fun, no matter how old you are.

This COULD be interesting...

This WILL be fun!

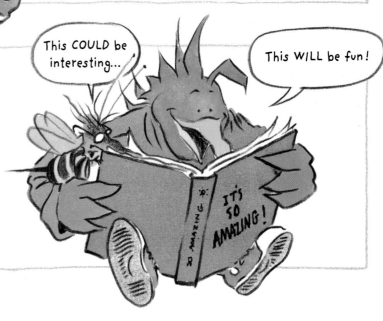

EGG + SPERM = BABY
Reproduction

When a new baby animal or plant is made, scientists call that "reproduction".
To reproduce means "to make again" – to make the same thing again.

Reproduction is how plants and animals make new plants and animals like themselves.

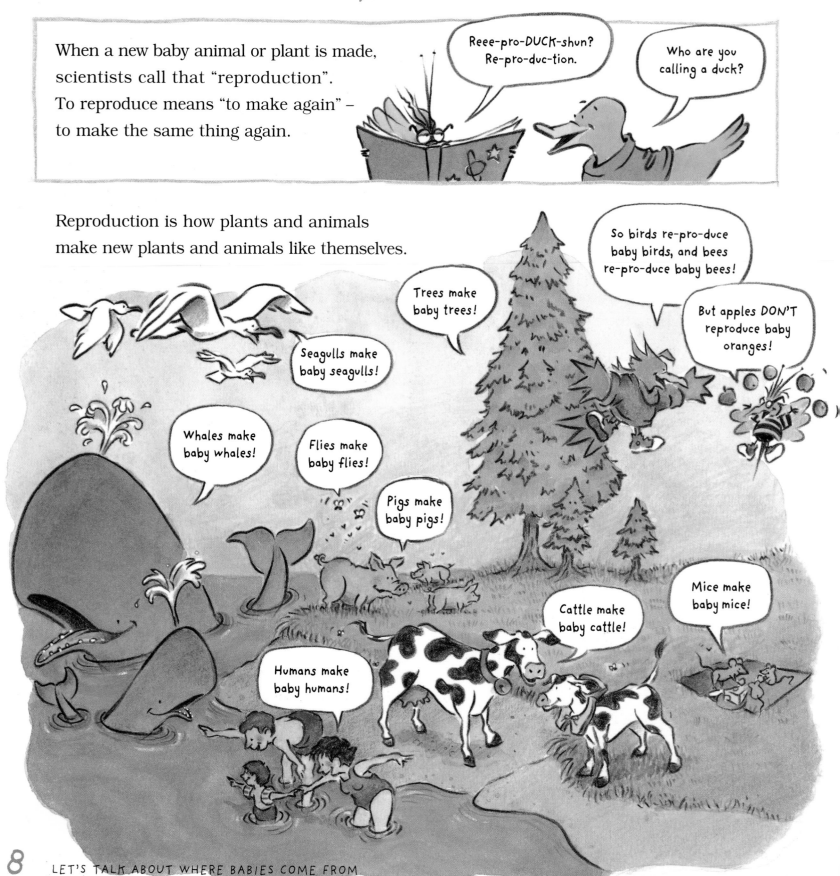

One fact about making a human baby is quite simple. It takes a sperm and an egg to make a baby.

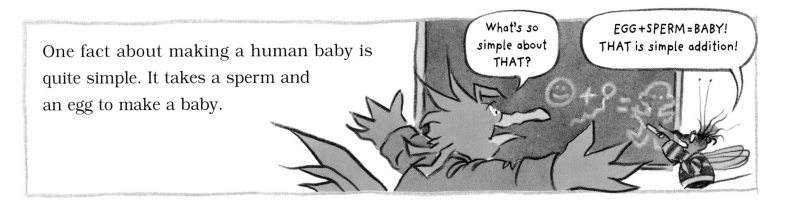

Sperm and eggs are cells. In fact, all plants and animals – including humans – are made up of cells. And the human body is made up of millions and millions and millions of cells.

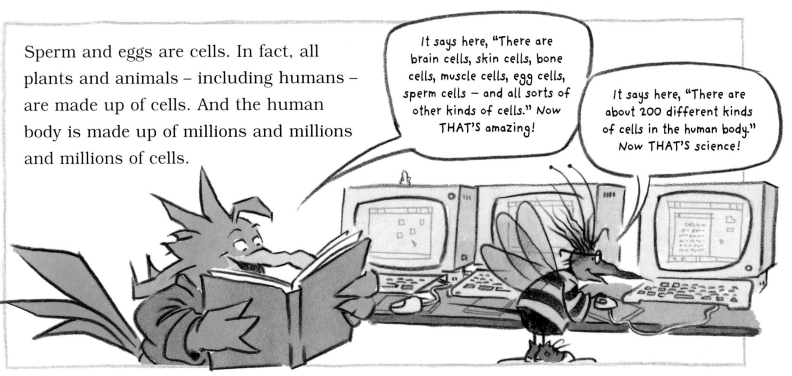

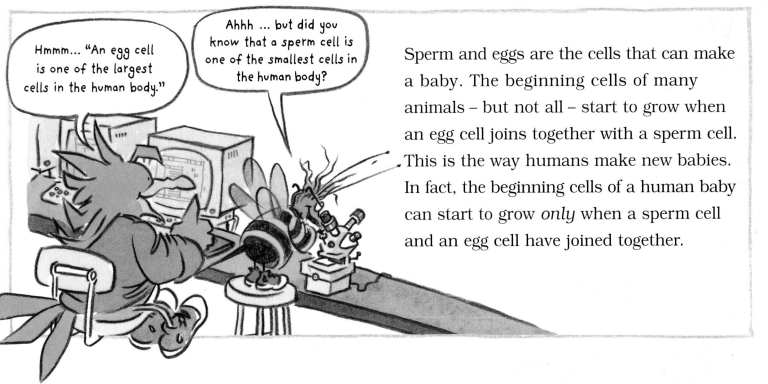

Sperm and eggs are the cells that can make a baby. The beginning cells of many animals – but not all – start to grow when an egg cell joins together with a sperm cell. This is the way humans make new babies. In fact, the beginning cells of a human baby can start to grow *only* when a sperm cell and an egg cell have joined together.

SAME AND DIFFERENT
Male – Female

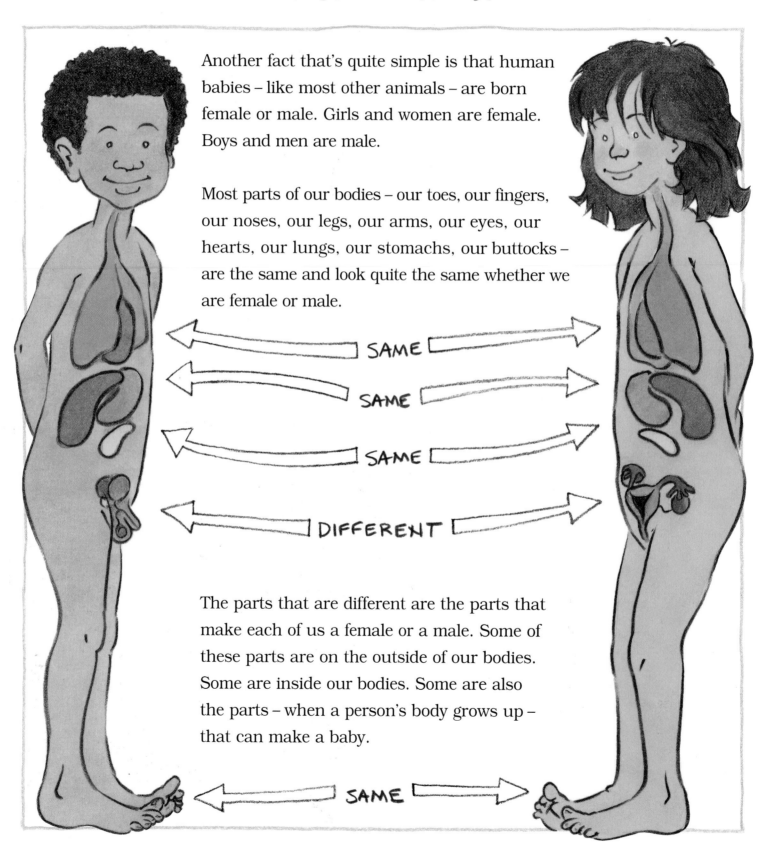

Another fact that's quite simple is that human babies – like most other animals – are born female or male. Girls and women are female. Boys and men are male.

Most parts of our bodies – our toes, our fingers, our noses, our legs, our arms, our eyes, our hearts, our lungs, our stomachs, our buttocks – are the same and look quite the same whether we are female or male.

SAME

SAME

SAME

DIFFERENT

The parts that are different are the parts that make each of us a female or a male. Some of these parts are on the outside of our bodies. Some are inside our bodies. Some are also the parts – when a person's body grows up – that can make a baby.

SAME

A male's sperm is needed to make a baby. Sperm are made in the male parts called "testicles". When a boy's body grows up, his two testicles will make an amazing amount of sperm – about one hundred million to three hundred million each day.

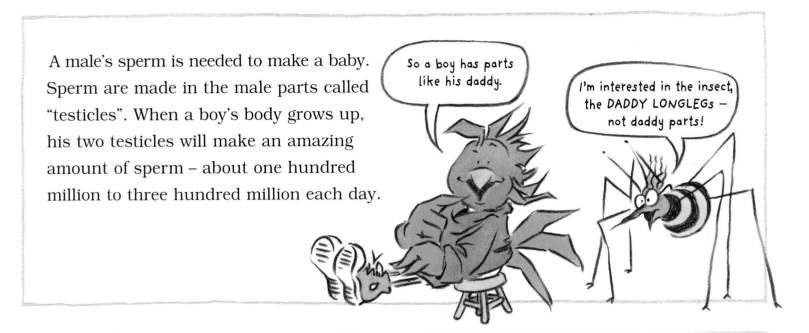

A female's egg is needed to make a baby. Eggs are stored inside the female parts called "ovaries". When a baby girl is born, her two ovaries have all the eggs – about one million to two million – she will ever need to make a baby.

Although every boy is born with the parts that will make millions of sperm, and every girl is born with the parts that store millions of eggs, those parts cannot make a baby until a child's body has grown up. And that time is called "puberty".

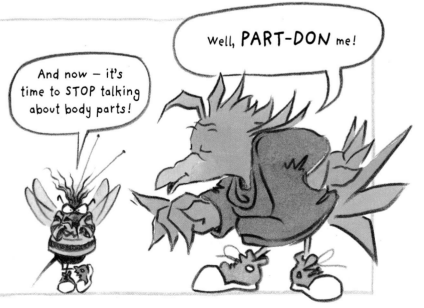

④

GROWING UP
Babies, Children, Teenagers, Grown-ups

You've been growing up since you were a tiny baby. But puberty is the time when a girl's body changes and becomes a woman's body, and when a boy's body changes and becomes a man's body.

You may even have noticed children who are going through puberty. Perhaps you have noticed an older brother or sister or cousin – or an older child in your school or who lives near you – whose body is beginning to change and look more and more like an adult's body.

During puberty, girls' and boys' bodies change in many ways. These changes do not happen all at once. For most children, these changes take place over a few years.

Since it takes a sperm and an egg to make a baby, a male and a female can *only* make a baby after puberty has begun. But most of the time, it's easier and healthier for people to wait to have a baby until they are older and have become grown-ups. That's because every baby needs a lot of love and care.

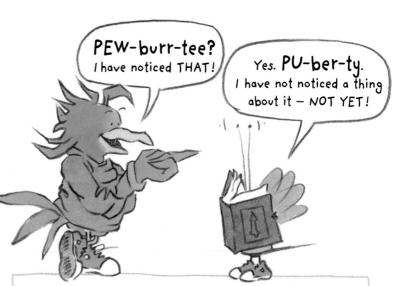

PEW-burr-tee? I have noticed THAT!

Yes. PU-ber-ty. I have not noticed a thing about it – NOT YET!

WHAT HAPPENS DURING PUBERTY?

- Girls *and* boys grow hair under their arms, on their arms and on their legs.

- Boys *and* girls sweat more.

- Some girls *and* some boys get spots on their face, chest and back.

- Boys' voices become deeper.

- Girls' hips grow wider and their breasts grow larger.

- Girls grow hair around the vulva – the area of soft skin between a female's legs.

- Boys grow hair on their upper lips and chests and at the base of the penis.

- Girls' ovaries start to send out eggs.

- Boys' testicles start to make sperm.

So first you're a baby, then you're a child, then you're a teenager and then you're a grown-up. That's a lot of growing up to do!

I like being a child. I'd like to stay being a child. Wouldn't you?

GROWING, GROWING, GROWING UP!

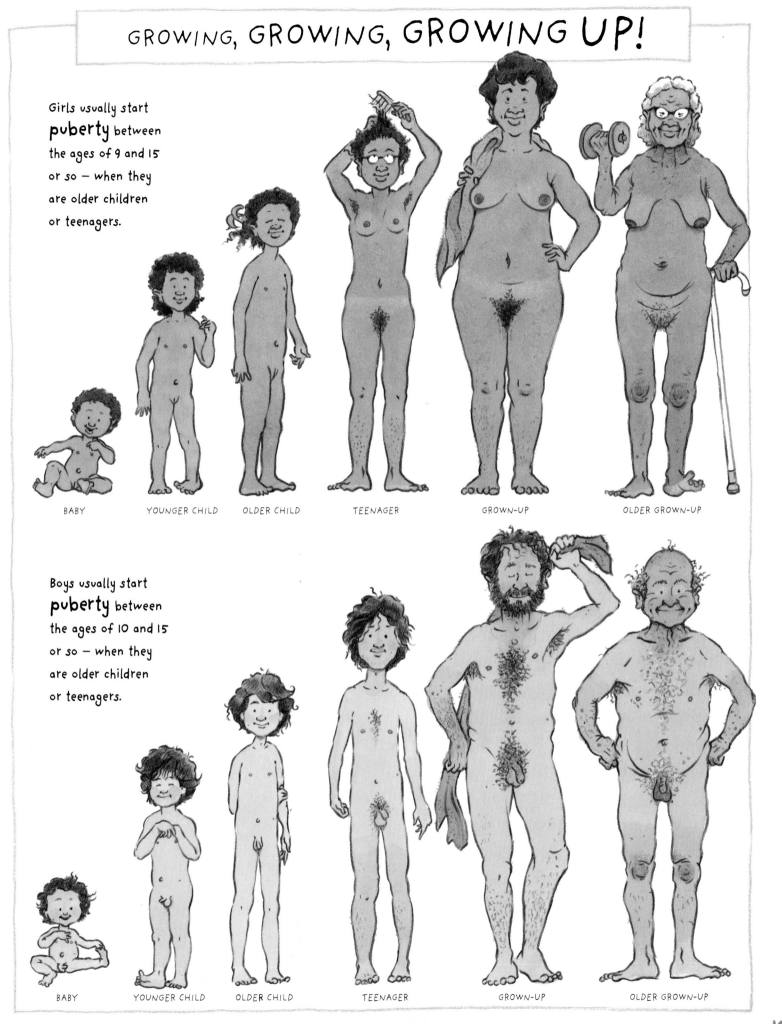

Girls usually start **puberty** between the ages of 9 and 15 or so — when they are older children or teenagers.

BABY   YOUNGER CHILD   OLDER CHILD   TEENAGER   GROWN-UP   OLDER GROWN-UP

Boys usually start **puberty** between the ages of 10 and 15 or so — when they are older children or teenagers.

BABY   YOUNGER CHILD   OLDER CHILD   TEENAGER   GROWN-UP   OLDER GROWN-UP

WHAT'S INSIDE? WHAT'S OUTSIDE?
Female Parts

Girls' bodies – even baby girls' bodies – and women's bodies all have female parts. They are the parts that can make a baby – but *not* until *after* puberty has begun.

The female parts that are INSIDE baby girls', girls' and women's bodies are below the tummy-button and under the stomach and intestines.

Most of the female parts on the OUTSIDE of baby girls', girls' and women's bodies are tucked between a female's legs.

A female's breasts are also on the OUTSIDE of her body. They grow larger *after* puberty has begun. And if and when a female has a baby, her breasts can make milk to feed the baby.

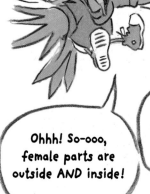

Ohhh! So-ooo, female parts are outside AND inside!

I don't care where they are — outside OR inside — as long as we stop TALKING and TALKING about them!

WHAT'S INSIDE?

The two OVARIES hold a female's eggs. The ovaries are about the size of grapes or marbles when a girl is young. During puberty, a girl's two ovaries grow to be about the size of large strawberries.

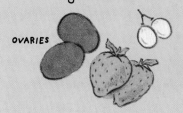

OVARIES

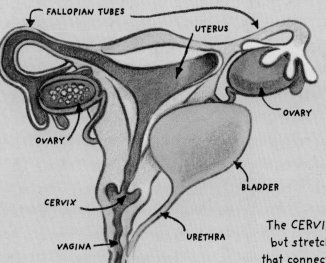

FALLOPIAN TUBES

UTERUS

OVARY

BLADDER

OVARY

CERVIX

URETHRA

VAGINA

The UTERUS is made of strong and stretchy muscles. It is about the size and shape of a small upside-down pear.

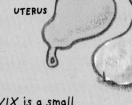

UTERUS

The FALLOPIAN TUBES are two narrow tubes whose flowerlike openings are next to the ovaries. Each tube is about as wide as a drinking straw. Each tube is connected to the uterus.

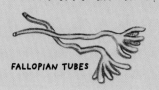

FALLOPIAN TUBES

The VAGINA is a small but stretchy passageway that leads from the uterus to a small opening between a female's legs.

The CERVIX is a small but stretchy opening that connects the uterus to the vagina.

The URETHRA is a narrow tube that leads from the bladder to another small opening between a female's legs. Both females *and* males have a urethra and a bladder.

WHAT'S OUTSIDE?

The area of soft skin between a female's legs is called the VULVA.

Inside the vulva are two folds of soft skin called the LABIA. The labia cover and protect the inner parts of the vulva.

The CLITORIS — a small bump of skin about the size of a pea — is at the front of the labia.

Two openings — THE OPENING TO THE URETHRA and THE OPENING TO THE VAGINA — are tucked inside the labia.

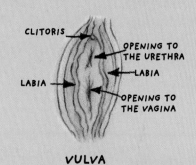

CLITORIS

OPENING TO THE URETHRA

LABIA

LABIA

OPENING TO THE VAGINA

VULVA

THE OPENING TO THE URETHRA is behind the clitoris. Urine — also called "wee" — leaves a female's body through the small opening to the urethra.

THE OPENING TO THE VAGINA is behind the opening to the urethra. When most babies are born, the baby comes out through the opening to the vagina.

Behind the labia is another small opening called the ANUS. Solid waste — also called "poo" — leaves a female's body through the anus. Both females *and* males have an anus.

In all, from front to back, there are three openings between a female's legs — the opening to her urethra, the opening to her vagina and her anus.

WHAT'S INSIDE?
WHAT'S OUTSIDE?
Male Parts

Boys' bodies – even baby boys' bodies – and men's bodies all have male parts. They are the parts that can make a baby – but *not* until *after* puberty has begun.

The male parts that are INSIDE baby boys', boys' and men's bodies are below the tummy-button and under the stomach and intestines.

The male parts on the OUTSIDE of baby boys', boys' and men's bodies hang between their legs.

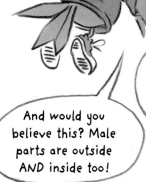

I don't care if they are outside OR inside — OR inside-out — as long as you stop TALKING about them!

And would you believe this? Male parts are outside AND inside too!

WHAT'S INSIDE?

The two TESTICLES make sperm after puberty has begun. The testicles are about the size of grapes or marbles when a boy is young. During puberty, a boy's two testicles grow to be the size of walnuts or very small balls. That's why some people call them "nuts" or "balls".

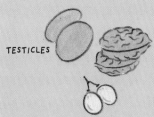

TESTICLES

The EPIDIDYMIS is a long, twisty, coiled tube. It is shaped somewhat like a telephone receiver, but smaller. Boys and men have two of these tubes. Each tube is connected to and wraps along the side of a testicle.

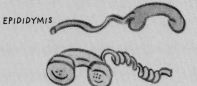

EPIDIDYMIS

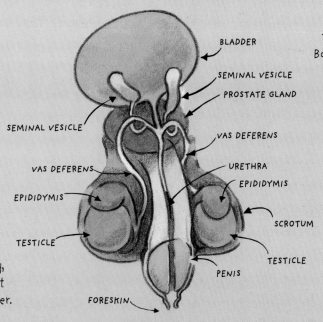

BLADDER
SEMINAL VESICLE
PROSTATE GLAND
SEMINAL VESICLE
VAS DEFERENS
VAS DEFERENS
URETHRA
EPIDIDYMIS
EPIDIDYMIS
SCROTUM
TESTICLE
TESTICLE
PENIS
FORESKIN

The PENIS is made of spongy tissue. Inside the penis, there is a narrow tube called the urethra.

The VAS DEFERENS is a long narrow tube that leads from the epididymis to the urethra. Boys and men have two of these tubes. They look like strands of cooked spaghetti.

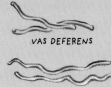

VAS DEFERENS

The SEMINAL VESICLES and PROSTATE GLAND are tucked along the side of the vas deferens.

The URETHRA is a narrow tube inside the penis that leads from the bladder to the small opening at the tip of the penis. Both males and females have a urethra and a bladder.

WHAT'S OUTSIDE?

The PENIS hangs in front of the scrotum. There is a small opening at the tip of the penis.

The SCROTUM is a sac of soft, squishy skin that covers and protects the two testicles. After puberty has begun, the scrotum keeps the testicles at just the right temperature to make sperm.

The FORESKIN is a layer of loose skin that covers the end of the penis.

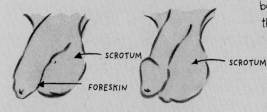

SCROTUM
FORESKIN
SCROTUM

UNCIRCUMCISED PENIS   CIRCUMCISED PENIS

Some male babies have the foreskin removed by a doctor or a specially trained religious person a few days after birth. This is called a "circumcision". Some male babies do not have the foreskin removed. Either way is perfectly normal.

Urine — also called "wee" — leaves a male's body through the small opening at the tip of the penis. After puberty has begun, sperm also leave through the tip of the penis. But urine and sperm do not leave the penis at the same time.

Behind the scrotum and penis is another small opening called the ANUS. Solid waste — also called "poo" — leaves a male's body through the anus. Both males and females have an anus.

In all, from front to back, there are two openings between a male's legs — the small opening at the tip of his penis and his anus.

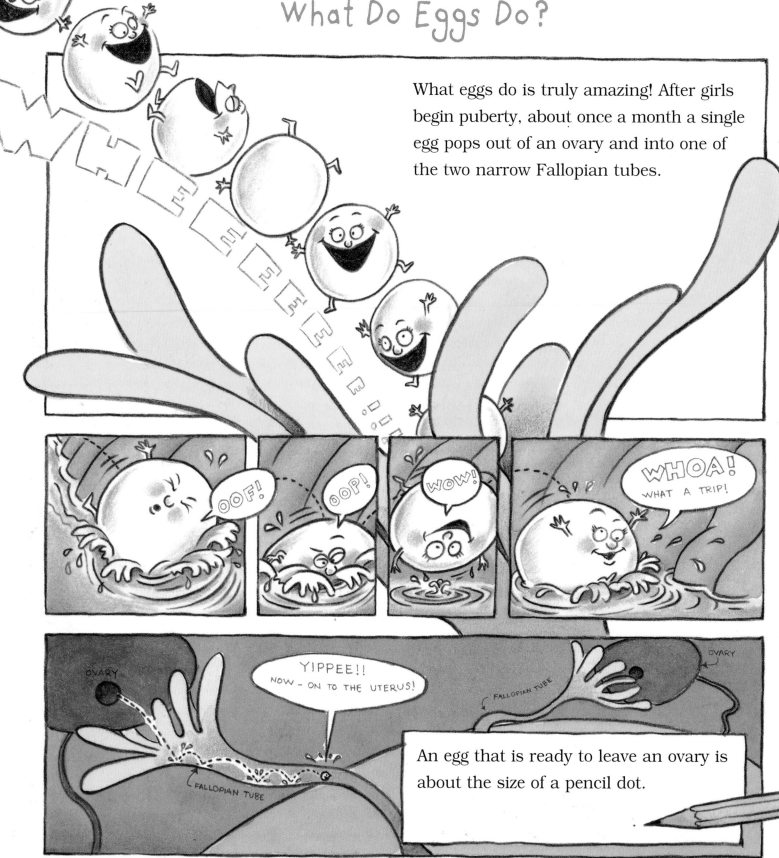

⑦ THE AMAZING EGG TRIP
What Do Eggs Do?

What eggs do is truly amazing! After girls begin puberty, about once a month a single egg pops out of an ovary and into one of the two narrow Fallopian tubes.

OOF!

OOP!

WOW!

WHOA! WHAT A TRIP!

YIPPEE!! NOW — ON TO THE UTERUS!

OVARY

FALLOPIAN TUBE

OVARY

FALLOPIAN TUBE

An egg that is ready to leave an ovary is about the size of a pencil dot.

When an egg meets and joins with a sperm …

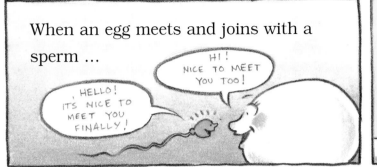

the united egg-and-sperm travels to the uterus where it can grow – over nine months – into a baby.

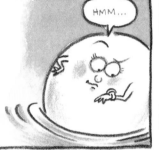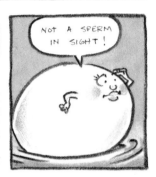

But most of the time, an egg does *not* meet a sperm. And if an egg does *not* meet a sperm, the beginning cells of a baby will *not* start to grow.

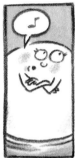

When an egg does *not* meet a sperm, the egg travels on to the uterus.

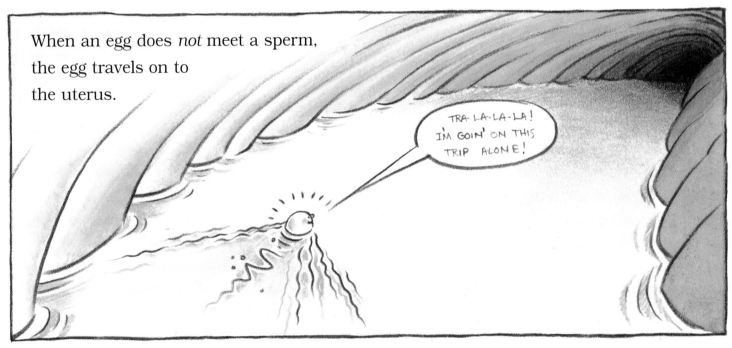

Then the egg breaks down and mixes with a small amount of blood from the uterus and flows out of a girl's or woman's body through her vagina.

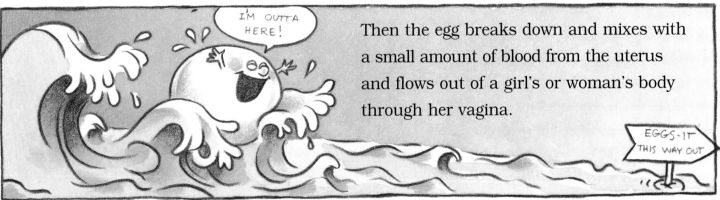

When the egg breaks down and leaves the uterus with the small amount of blood, this is called "menstruation", or "menstruating", or "having a period".

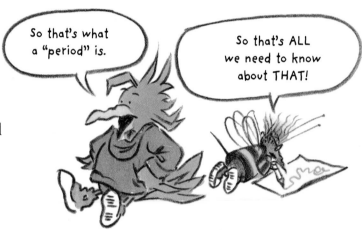

Men-stroo-a-shun?

Say a word 3 times and it's yours! Men-stru-a-tion! Men-struation! Menstruation!

The blood that flows out of the uterus and through the vagina does *not* come from a cut. And it does *not* appear because a girl or woman is sick or has been hurt. The blood comes from the soft lining of the uterus. And the lining and blood leave the uterus with the egg – and leave a girl's or woman's body through her vagina.

So that's what a "period" is.

So that's ALL we need to know about THAT!

The blood from a period passes through the vagina and leaves a girl's or woman's body through the opening to her vagina. But urine, also called "wee", flows from the bladder – where it is stored – and flows through a passageway called the urethra. Urine leaves a girl's or woman's body through the opening to her urethra.

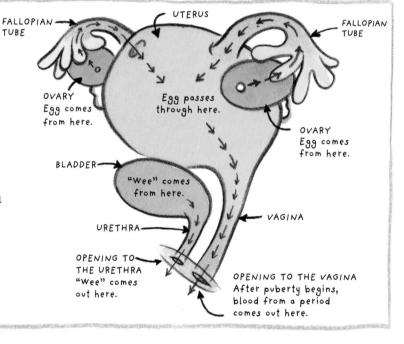

FALLOPIAN TUBE

UTERUS

FALLOPIAN TUBE

OVARY
Egg comes from here.

Egg passes through here.

OVARY
Egg comes from here.

BLADDER

"Wee" comes from here.

URETHRA

VAGINA

OPENING TO THE URETHRA
"Wee" comes out here.

OPENING TO THE VAGINA
After puberty begins, blood from a period comes out here.

Each month, another egg is ready to leave one of the ovaries and a new lining is made. The lining is needed only when a united egg-and-sperm cell – the beginning cells of a baby – starts to grow in the uterus.

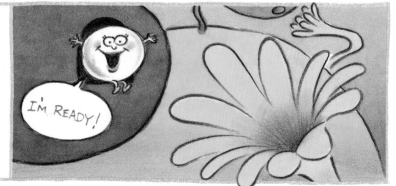

I'M READY!

During a period, girls and women wear a soft, cottonlike "pad" inside their underpants, or a roll of cottonlike material that is shaped to fit inside the vagina. This is called a "tampon". The pad or tampon soaks up the small amount of blood so that it will not get on their clothes.

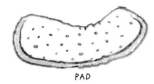

PAD

TAMPON

I've heard ALL about THAT!

I've heard E-NOUGH!

Girls do *not* begin to menstruate – to have periods – until *after* puberty has begun, sometime between the ages of nine and fifteen or so. When a woman becomes pregnant, her periods stop. But they start again after her baby is born. When women are about fifty years old they stop having periods and do not have them again. That's because their ovaries stop sending out eggs.

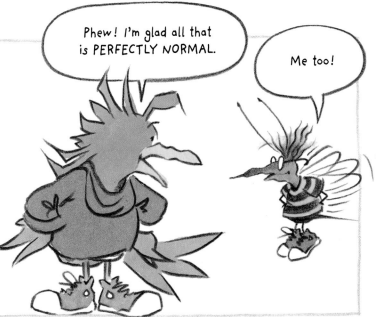

Phew! I'm glad all that is PERFECTLY NORMAL.

Me too!

It's so amazing that if an egg meets a sperm, the beginning cells of a baby can start to grow! It's also amazing that if an egg does not meet a sperm, the egg travels out of the female's body, and the next month, another egg is ready to leave one of the ovaries!

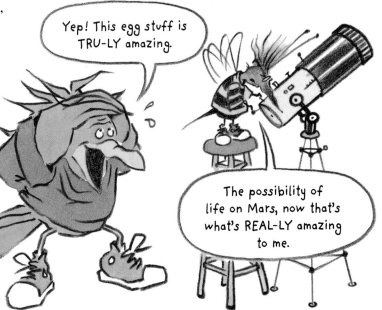

Yep! This egg stuff is TRU-LY amazing.

The possibility of life on Mars, now that's what's REAL-LY amazing to me.

⑧ THE AMAZING SPERM TRIP
What Do Sperm Do?

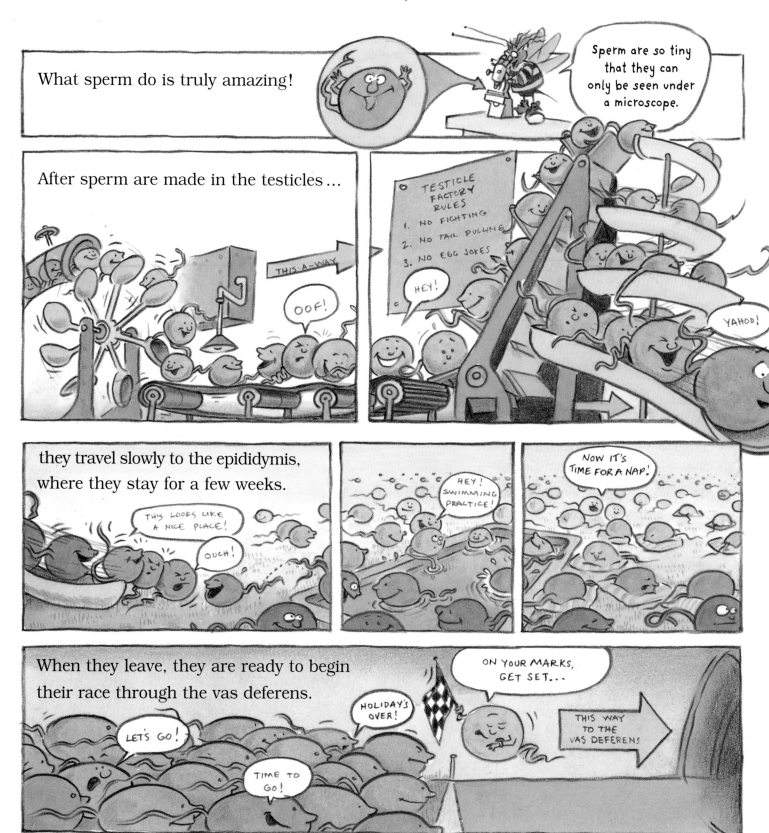

What sperm do is truly amazing!

Sperm are so tiny that they can only be seen under a microscope.

After sperm are made in the testicles ...

THIS-A-WAY

OOF!

TESTICLE FACTORY RULES
1. NO FIGHTING
2. NO TAIL PULLING
3. NO EGG JOKES

HEY!

YAHOO!

they travel slowly to the epididymis, where they stay for a few weeks.

THIS LOOKS LIKE A NICE PLACE!

OUCH!

HEY! SWIMMING PRACTICE!

NOW IT'S TIME FOR A NAP!

When they leave, they are ready to begin their race through the vas deferens.

LET'S GO!

HOLIDAY'S OVER!

TIME TO GO!

ON YOUR MARKS, GET SET...

THIS WAY TO THE VAS DEFERENS

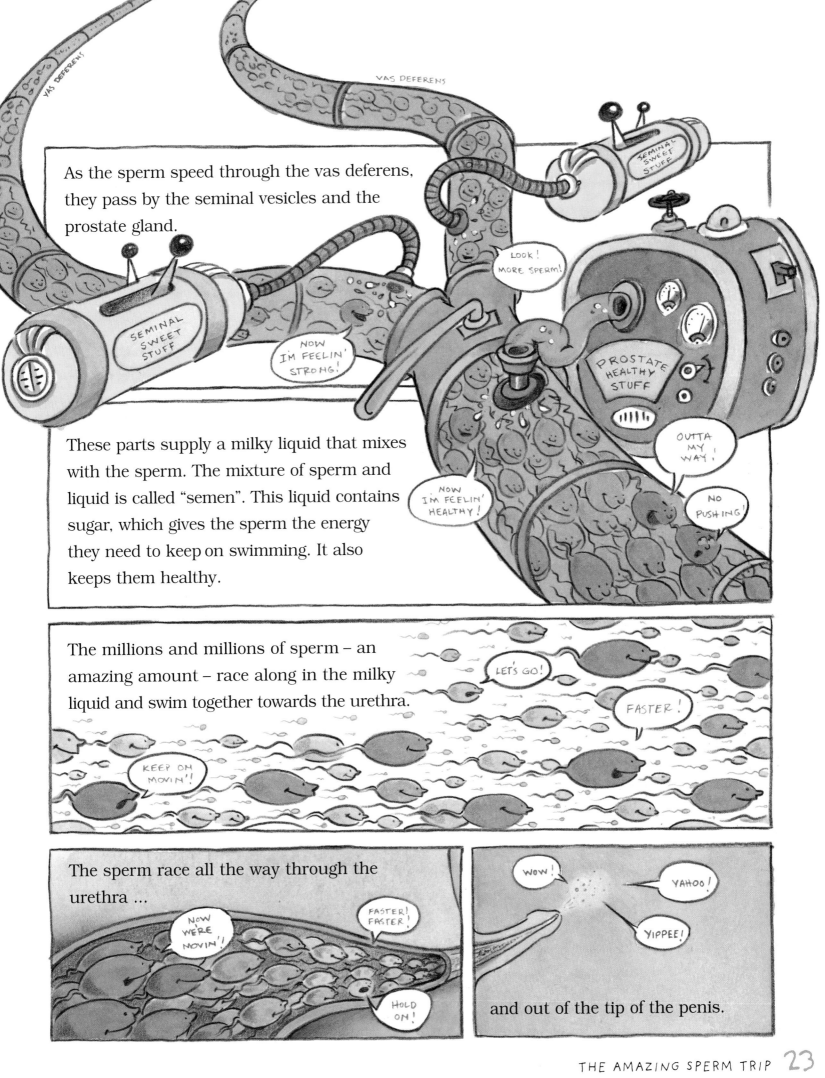

As the sperm speed through the vas deferens, they pass by the seminal vesicles and the prostate gland.

These parts supply a milky liquid that mixes with the sperm. The mixture of sperm and liquid is called "semen". This liquid contains sugar, which gives the sperm the energy they need to keep on swimming. It also keeps them healthy.

The millions and millions of sperm – an amazing amount – race along in the milky liquid and swim together towards the urethra.

The sperm race all the way through the urethra ...

and out of the tip of the penis.

Sometimes the penis becomes stiff and larger, and stands out from the body. This is called "having an erection". After puberty begins, semen can – but does not always – come out of the tip of the penis during an erection. When this happens, it is called an "ejaculation". This is how sperm leave the penis.

A boy's testicles do *not* make sperm until *after* puberty begins. That's why sperm do *not* come out of the tip of a young boy's penis. But older boys' and men's testicles *do* make sperm and continue to make sperm into old age.

And if just one of those sperm travelling along in the semen meets an egg, the beginning cells of a baby can start to grow.

Having an erection is perfectly healthy and perfectly normal at any age. Baby boys, boys, teenage boys, men and old men have erections. Even before boy babies are born, they have erections inside the uterus.

Sometimes when a boy who has begun puberty – or a teenage boy or a man – has a dream, he may have an erection, and semen may come out of the tip of his penis. This is called "having a wet dream". Boys do *not* begin to have wet dreams until *after* puberty begins – sometime between the ages of ten and fifteen or so.

Phew! I'm glad all that is PERFECTLY NORMAL.

Me too!

Urine, also called "wee", flows from the bladder – where it is stored – and out of boys' and men's bodies through the urethra and out of the tip of the penis. But urine *does not* and *cannot* leave the penis at the same time as semen. That's because during an ejaculation, muscles at the top of the penis tighten and stop the urine from leaving.

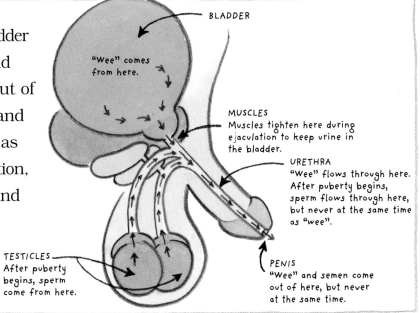

BLADDER

"Wee" comes from here.

MUSCLES
Muscles tighten here during ejaculation to keep urine in the bladder.

URETHRA
"Wee" flows through here. After puberty begins, sperm flows through here, but never at the same time as "wee".

TESTICLES
After puberty begins, sperm come from here.

PENIS
"Wee" and semen come out of here, but never at the same time.

It's so amazing that if a sperm meets an egg, the beginning cells of a baby can start to grow! It's also amazing that millions of new sperm are made every day and that sperm can swim so fast and so far!

Yep! This sperm stuff is TRU-LY amazing!

The fact that humans have walked on the moon, now that's what's REAL-LY amazing to me.

WHAT'S SEX?

Female or Male – Loving – Making Love – Making a Baby

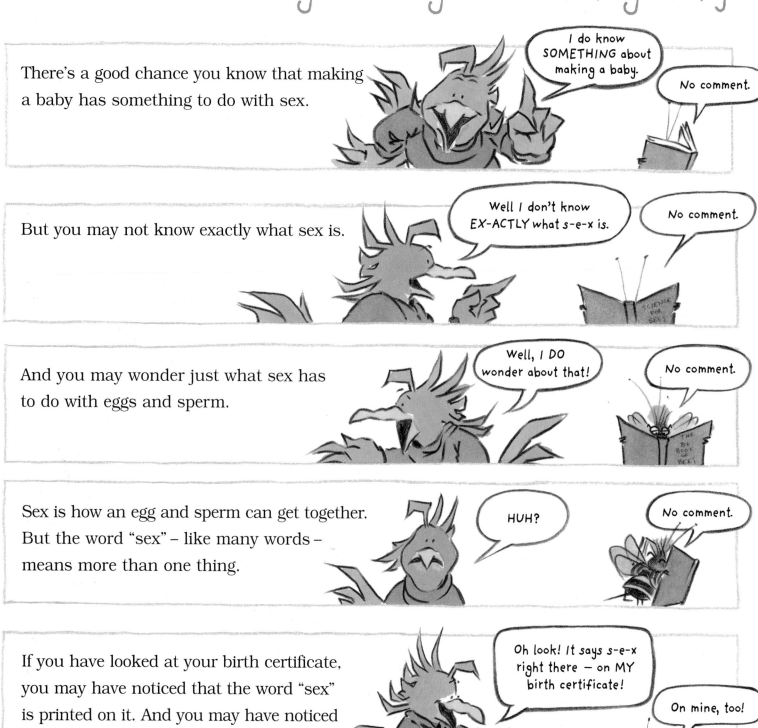

There's a good chance you know that making a baby has something to do with sex.

I do know SOMETHING about making a baby.

No comment.

But you may not know exactly what sex is.

Well I don't know EX-ACTLY what s-e-x is.

No comment.

And you may wonder just what sex has to do with eggs and sperm.

Well, I DO wonder about that!

No comment.

Sex is how an egg and sperm can get together. But the word "sex" – like many words – means more than one thing.

HUH?

No comment.

If you have looked at your birth certificate, you may have noticed that the word "sex" is printed on it. And you may have noticed that the word "female" or "male", or the letter "F" or "M", is typed or written next to the word "sex".

Oh look! It says s-e-x right there – on MY birth certificate!

On mine, too!

Your birth certificate is a record of the day and year of your birth. It's also a record of the city or town and the country you were born in, and of your parents' names. And it's also a record of whether you were born a member of the female sex or a member of the male sex.

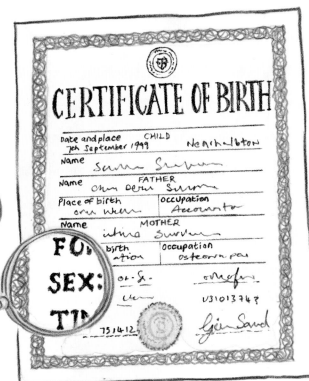

But that's not all s-e-x means!

I can s-p-e-l-l, you know!

What sex you are – female or male – is also called your "gender". When the word "sex" is used in this way, it means whether a person is a female or a male – a girl or a boy, a woman or a man. When a new baby is born – and sometimes even before birth – one of the first questions almost everyone asks is, "Is it a girl or a boy?" People always want to know the sex, or gender, of a new baby.

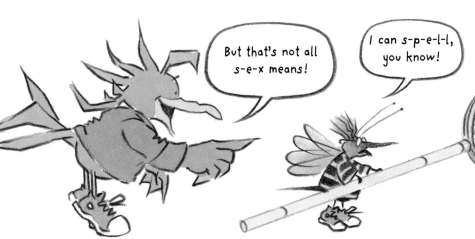

It's a boy!

A girl?

Boy?

Girl?

?!

So what sex is it?

Sex can be about other things, too – like loving, caring and touching. Sex can also be about making a baby. When a woman and a man want to make a baby, they hug and cuddle and kiss and feel very loving, and get very close to each other – so close that the man's penis goes inside the woman's vagina. When this happens, it is called "sexual intercourse".

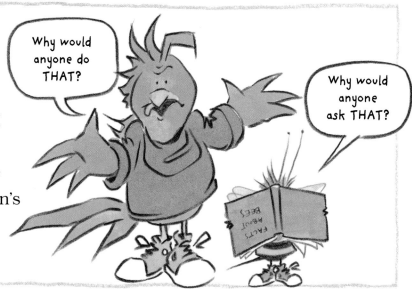

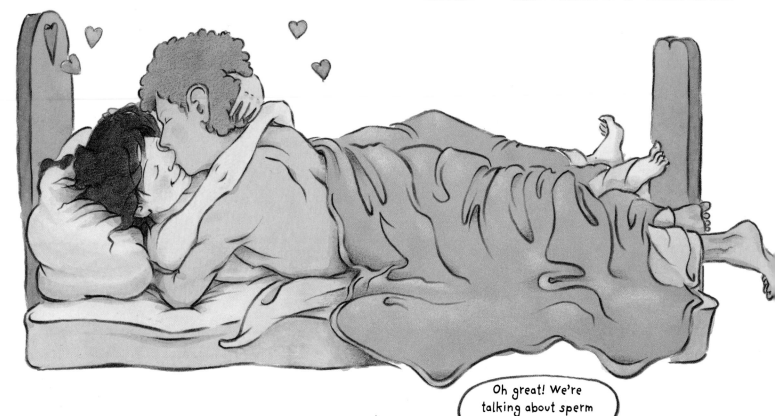

During sexual intercourse, millions of tiny sperm swim from the man's penis into the woman's vagina. And if just one of those sperm meets and joins together with an egg in one of the Fallopian tubes, the beginning cells of a baby can start to grow.

Some people call sexual intercourse "sex" or "having sex". When people grow up, having sex is one way to show their love for each other. That's why some people call sexual intercourse "making love". Grown-ups also make love when they are not planning to make a baby because it can feel good to be so close to each other.

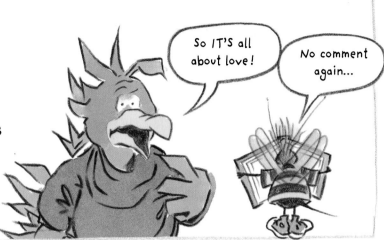

Sexual intercourse may seem gross or nice, scary or funny, weird or cool – or even unbelievable to you. But when two people care for each other, sexual intercourse is very loving. Children are much too young to have sexual intercourse.

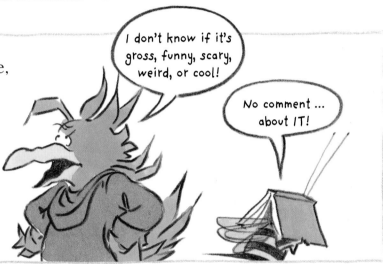

Loving and taking good care of a baby and a child take a lot of time and work. That's why it makes good sense for people to wait to have a baby until they have had time to grow up and are ready to become parents.

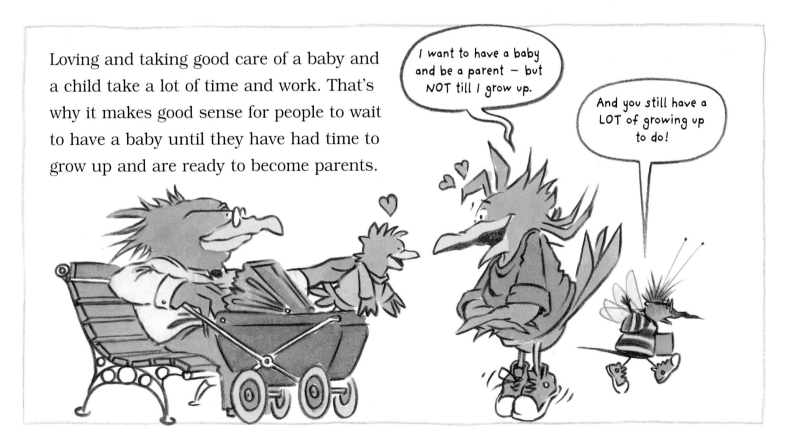

WHAT'S LOVE ?

Lots of Kinds of Love

When you like someone very much and have warm and good and loving feelings for that person, that's called "love". There are times when love and sex go together. But love and sex do not always go together. Sometimes people just love each other.

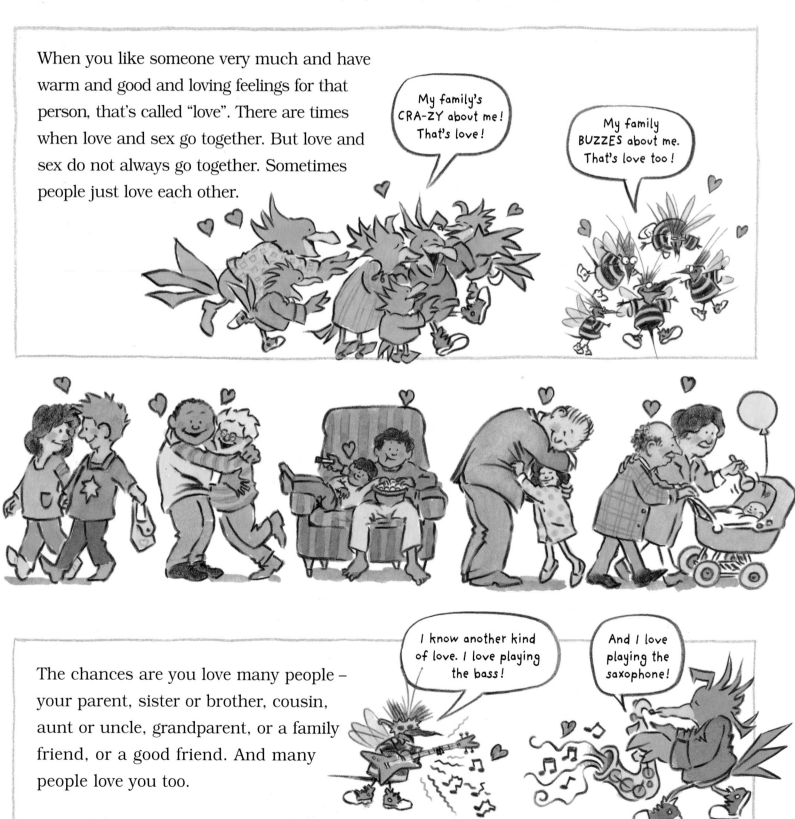

My family's CRA-ZY about me! That's love!

My family BUZZES about me. That's love too!

The chances are you love many people – your parent, sister or brother, cousin, aunt or uncle, grandparent, or a family friend, or a good friend. And many people love you too.

I know another kind of love. I love playing the bass!

And I love playing the saxophone!

You may have a best friend – or a group of friends – whom you love to be with and who love to be with you. If you have a pet – a cat or a dog or a fish or a guinea pig or a terrapin – you may also love your pet. You may also love a favourite cuddly toy. These kinds of love are not the same as "making love".

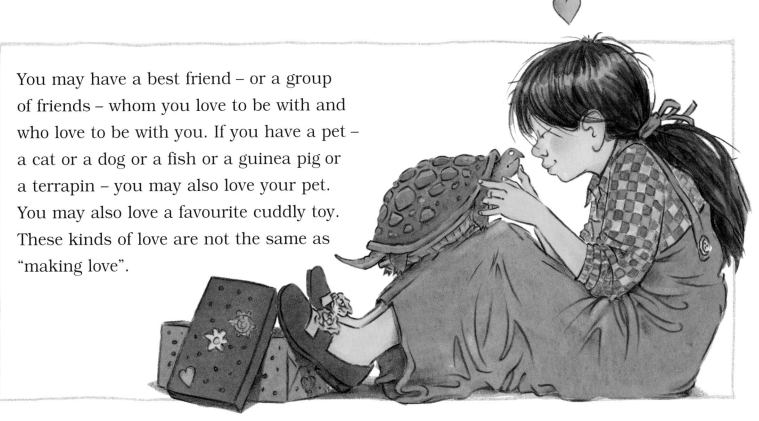

There are lots of kinds of love – like love between a parent and child, love between friends, love between children, love between teenagers and love between grown-ups. There can be love between a female and a male, or a male and a male, or a female and a female.

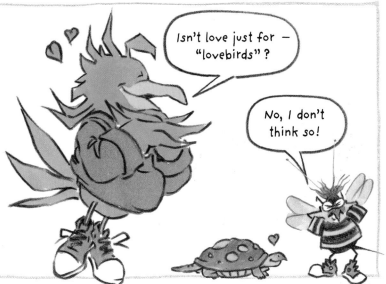

Isn't love just for – "lovebirds"?

No, I don't think so!

You may have heard the words "straight", "gay", and "lesbian". You may know – or you may wonder – what these words mean or what they have to do with love. You may have also heard the words "heterosexual" and "homosexual". Although these two words have the word "sex" in them, they can also be about love.

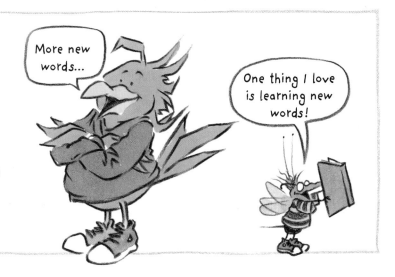

More new words...

One thing I love is learning new words!

Here's what the words "heterosexual" and "homosexual" mean.

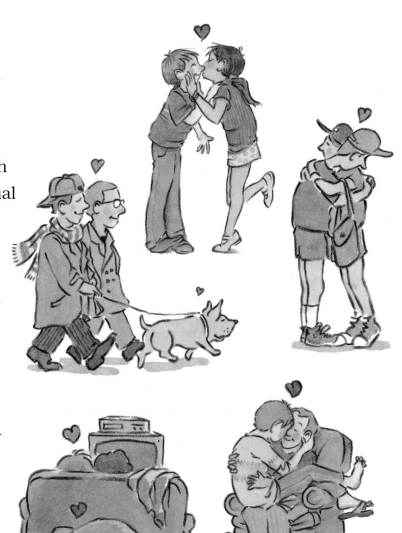

A female and a male who are sexually attracted to and who may fall in love with each other are called "heterosexual". A heterosexual person is sexually attracted – like a magnet – to the *other* sex or gender.

A female who is sexually attracted to and who may fall in love with another female is called "homosexual". A male who is sexually attracted to and who may fall in love with another male is also called "homosexual". A homosexual person is sexually attracted – like a magnet – to the *same* sex or gender.

The word "straight" is another name for a heterosexual male or female. The word "gay" is another name for a homosexual male or female. And the word "lesbian" is another name for a homosexual female.

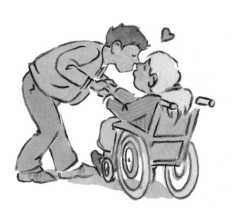

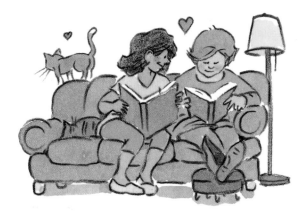

A person's daily life – having friends, having fun, going to work, being a mum or dad, loving another person – is mostly the same whether a person is straight or gay.

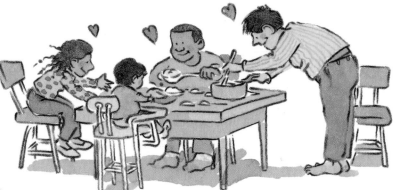

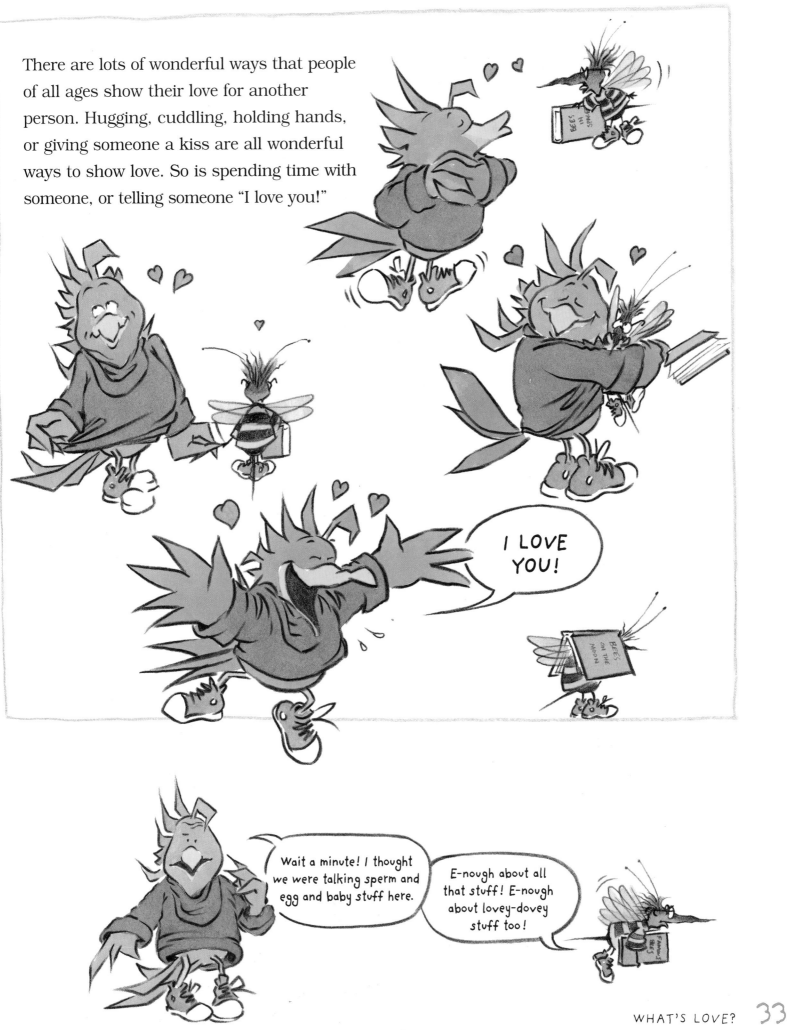

There are lots of wonderful ways that people of all ages show their love for another person. Hugging, cuddling, holding hands, or giving someone a kiss are all wonderful ways to show love. So is spending time with someone, or telling someone "I love you!"

THE BIG RACE!
Sperm and Egg Meet

It takes only one egg and one sperm to make a baby.

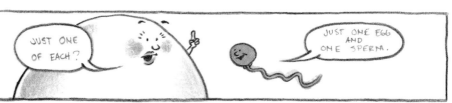

When a man and a woman have sexual intercourse, millions of tiny sperm travelling along in the semen race out of the tip of the man's penis and quickly swim into the woman's vagina.

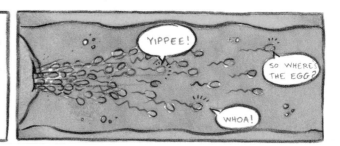

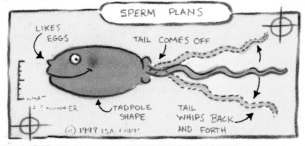

Sperm are shaped like tadpoles. Their long tails are what make them such speedy swimmers. When scientists watch sperm swim under a microscope, they can actually see the sperm's tails whipping and lashing back and forth.

After the sperm swim through the vagina, they race through a narrow opening called the cervix and into the uterus.

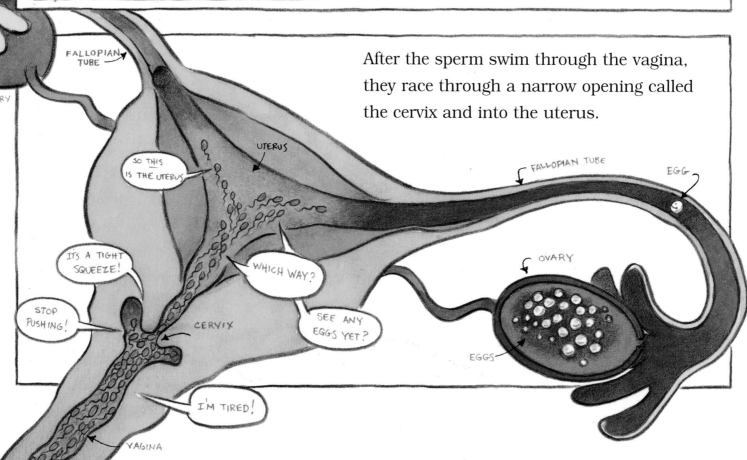

Then the sperm swim through the uterus and into the two narrow Fallopian tubes. If an egg has left an ovary and is in one of the Fallopian tubes, that's where a sperm can meet an egg.

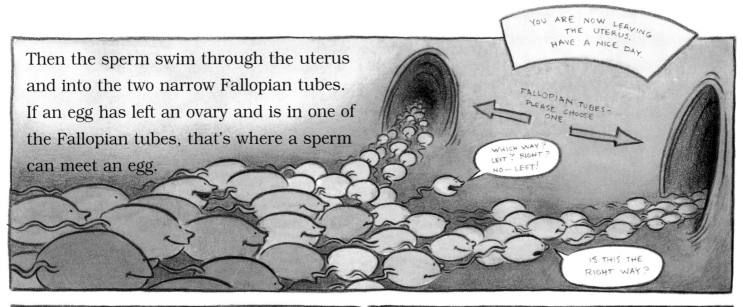

It usually takes several hours for the millions of sperm to swim all the way to the Fallopian tubes.

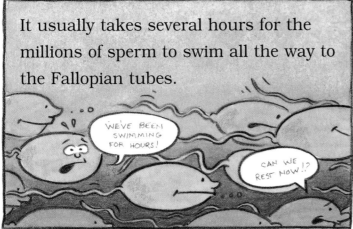

Usually only about two hundred sperm – out of the millions of sperm – swim to and get close to an egg.

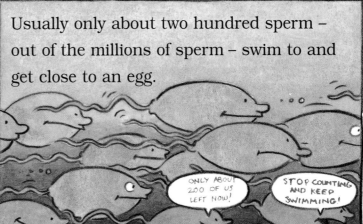

Scientists have discovered that if an egg is in one of the tubes, a chemical in the liquid around the egg attracts one sperm out of the two hundred sperm – just like a magnet.

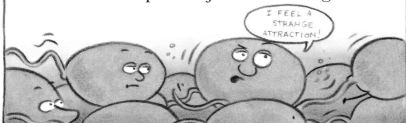

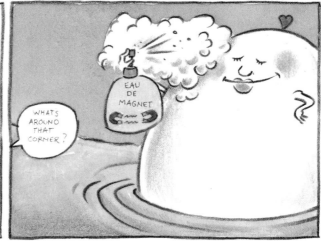

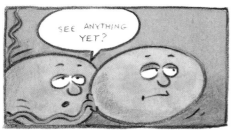

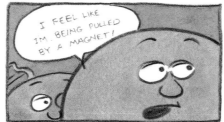

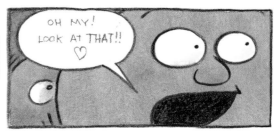

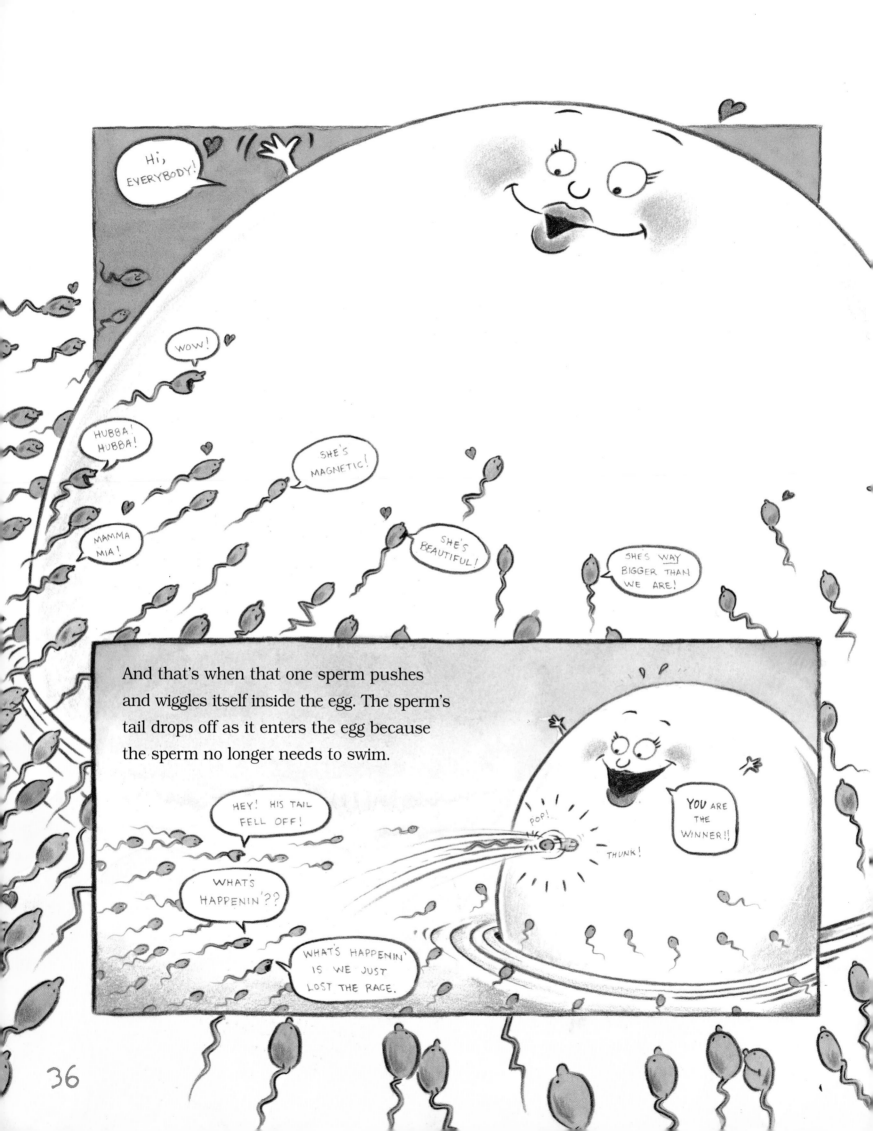

And that's when that one sperm pushes and wiggles itself inside the egg. The sperm's tail drops off as it enters the egg because the sperm no longer needs to swim.

The egg then closes up and does not let any of the other sperm enter.

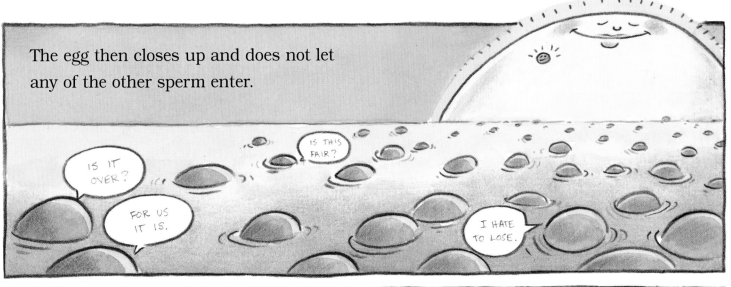

The moment a single sperm pushes itself inside the egg, the sperm and egg become one cell – the beginning cell of a baby.
The united sperm-and-egg is now called a fertilized egg cell, or a "zygote".

As the united cell travels through the Fallopian tube, it divides over and over again and becomes a ball of cells.

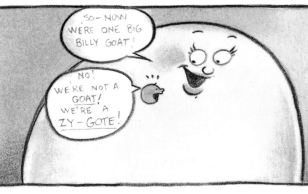

And after travelling through the tube for about five to seven days ...

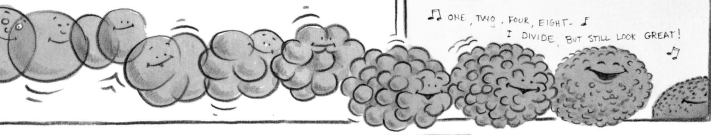

the ball of cells finally reaches the uterus. By this time, it has about one hundred cells.

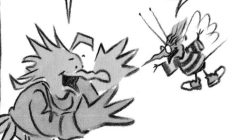

Sometimes when people want to have a baby, the egg cell and sperm cell are not able to meet. That's when some people choose to adopt a baby or child. And that's when some people use ways other than sexual intercourse for an egg cell and a sperm cell to meet. In fact, scientists have worked out several ways for an egg cell and a sperm cell to meet.

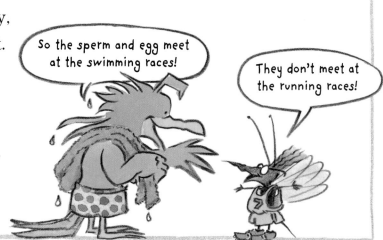

Doctors can place sperm into the vagina or the uterus with a syringe – a tube like an eyedropper.

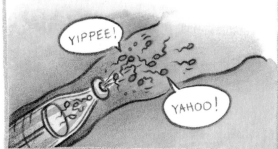

The sperm can then swim to the Fallopian tubes where a sperm can meet and join with an egg ...

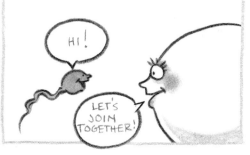

and travel to the uterus where the beginning cells of a baby can start to grow.

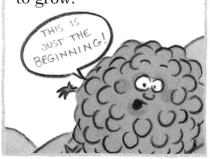

Or doctors can put an egg and a sperm in a special laboratory dish where the egg and sperm can meet and join together.

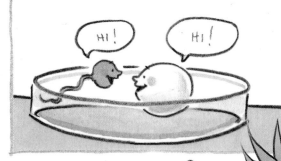

After they have joined, the doctor uses a syringe to place the united egg-and-sperm cell into the uterus ...

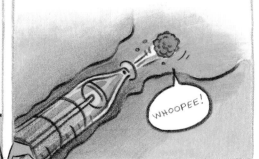

where the beginning cells of a baby can start to grow.

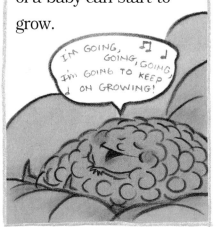

There are times when a man and a woman have sexual intercourse, but do not wish to make a baby. Scientists have invented ways called "contraception" or "birth control" that can stop a sperm and egg from meeting. And if a sperm and egg do not meet, the beginning cells of a baby cannot start to grow.

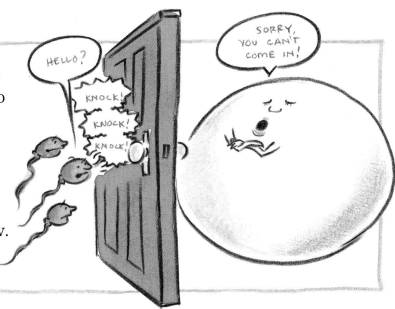

There are many kinds of contraception. One kind is a pill a woman can take. These pills can stop the ovaries from sending out an egg. A "condom" is another kind of birth control. A condom fits over the penis and can catch sperm before it can meet the egg. A condom can also stop people from getting or passing on infections like HIV – the infection that causes AIDS – during sexual intercourse.

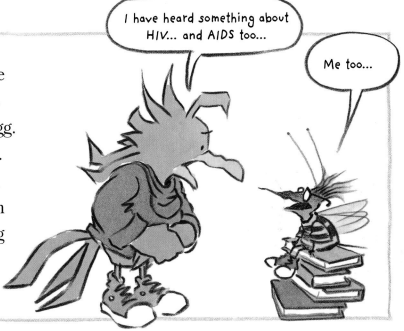

The only sure way for people *not* to get an infection from sex or *not* to have a baby is *not* to have sexual intercourse. And that is called "abstinence". Abstinence and birth control can help people choose whether or not to have a baby, or how many children to have, or when to have a baby.

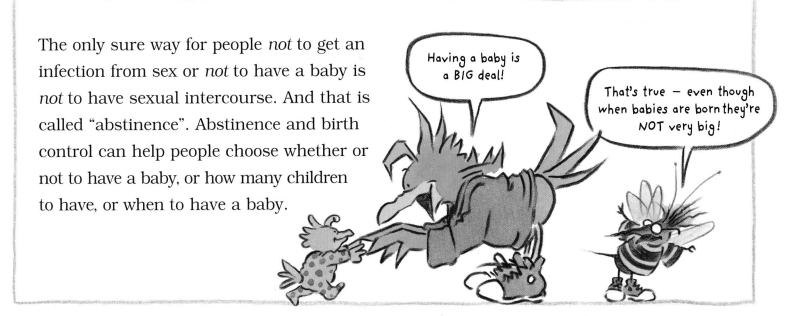

A WARM AND COSY WOMB
Pregnancy

It's so amazing that a tiny ball of cells can grow into a whole new person – a baby! But it can. Once the ball of cells arrives inside the uterus, it plants itself in the soft lining of the uterus.

It's so amazing that over nine months those cells will divide billions and billions of times to grow and become a baby! It takes a lot of time and growing to become a baby.

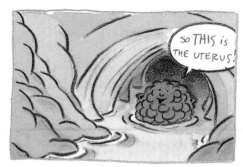

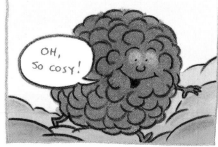

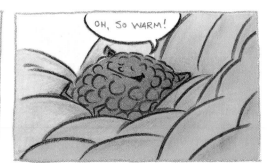

A woman is "pregnant" once the ball of cells starts to grow in the lining of her uterus. Now the ball of cells is called an "embryo". By three months, an embryo is called a "fetus". It is called a fetus until it is ready to be born.

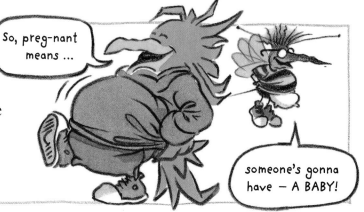

As a fetus grows bigger, the uterus gets bigger and stretches wide – like a balloon – to make more room. When a woman is pregnant, her uterus stretches from the size of a small pear to about the size of a watermelon. After eight or nine months of growing, the fetus moves around less because there's less room inside the uterus. After the baby is born, its mother's uterus shrinks back to its usual shape and size.

"Pregnancy" is the time it takes for an embryo to become a fetus and for a fetus to be born. Then it's a baby! A lot of children – and even some grown-ups – think that a fetus grows in its mother's stomach. A fetus does not grow in the stomach. A fetus grows in the uterus. Some people call the fetus "a growing baby".

WHERE DOES THE FOOD GO?

The food goes to the stomach. Inside the stomach, chemical juices break down the foods we eat and the liquids we drink and change them into very, very tiny bits.

WHERE DOES THE FETUS GROW?

A fetus grows in the uterus — a special, soft, warm, cosy, and safe place inside its mother's body below her tummy-button. The uterus is also called the "womb".

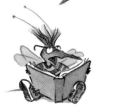

So the fetus doesn't grow where the pizza goes! Not in the stomach! That would be to-ooo messy!

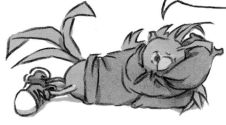

The uterus sounds like a warm and cosy womb for a nap! Get it? Got it? Womb? Room?

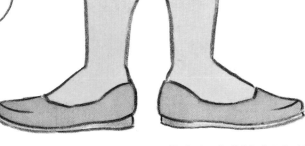

STOMACH

UTERUS

PIZZA

There are times when a pregnancy ends without warning – before an embryo or fetus is big enough and healthy enough to live outside the uterus. When this happens, it is called a "miscarriage". Most women who have had a miscarriage can become pregnant again and give birth to a strong and healthy baby.

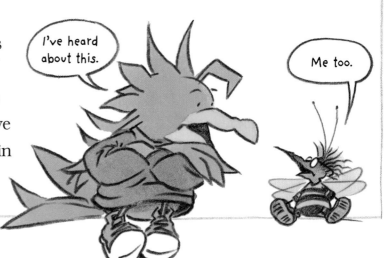

And there are times when a woman becomes pregnant and then chooses not to stay pregnant. She may then choose to have an "abortion". An abortion is a medical way to end a pregnancy. Most women who have had an abortion can become pregnant again and give birth to a strong and healthy baby.

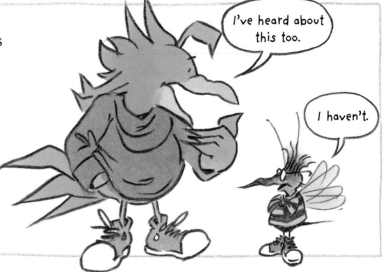

And there are times when a woman who is pregnant chooses not to bring up her baby. She may choose to stay pregnant and make a plan for her baby to be adopted. And when her baby is born, the baby can be adopted by a family who can love, care for and bring up that baby.

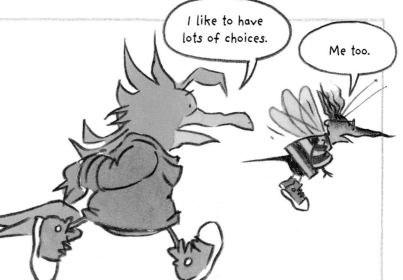

HOW LONG UNTIL IT'S A BABY?
Pregnancy

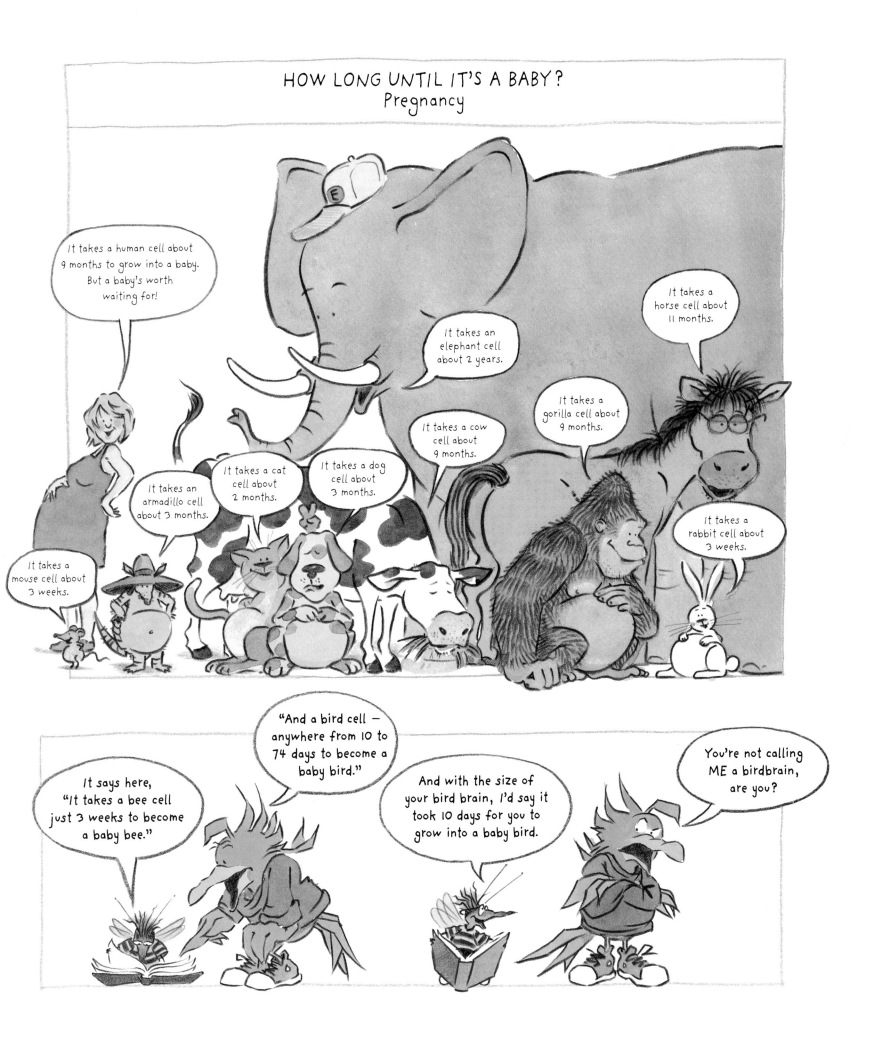

BALL OF CELLS TO BABY
9 Months of Growing

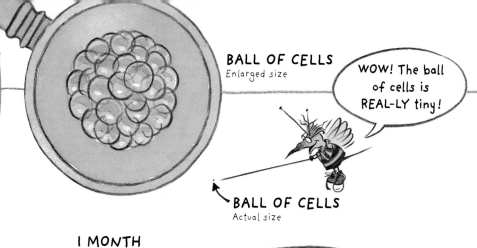

BALL OF CELLS
Enlarged size

WOW! The ball of cells is REAL-LY tiny!

BALL OF CELLS
Actual size

A pregnancy begins when the **BALL OF CELLS** plants itself in the lining of the uterus and becomes an embryo. By now, it has about 100 cells and is about the size of a pin point.

I MONTH
Actual size

I MONTH
Enlarged size

By **I MONTH,** an embryo is about the size of a tomato seed. Its backbone has begun to grow and its heart has begun to beat.

I 1/2 MONTHS
Actual size

By **I 1/2 MONTHS,** an embryo is about the size of a currant. The very beginnings of its arms, legs, fingers, toes, ears, eyes, nose and lips have begun to form.

I 1/2 MONTHS
Enlarged size

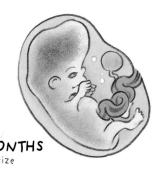

6 MONTHS
Actual size

By **2 MONTHS,** an embryo is about the size of a peach stone. By now, its fingers, toes, ears, eyes, nose and lips show. And its eyelids have begun to form.

2 MONTHS
Actual size

By **3 MONTHS,** when an embryo has become a fetus, it is about the size of a large peach. The parts that make a fetus male or female have formed. Fingernails and toenails have begun to grow. A fetus's body begins to be covered by soft fuzzy hair called "lanugo", and a slippery whitish coating called "vernix". The hair and coating protect a fetus from the water it floats in.

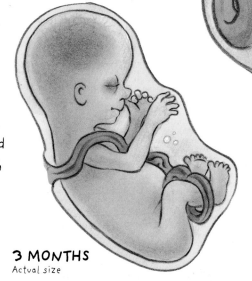

3 MONTHS
Actual size

By **6 MONTHS,** a fetus is about the size of a coconut. Eyebrows and eyelashes have grown. Some hair may have started to grow on its head. And its lungs have begun to practise breathing movements even though a fetus cannot breathe on its own.

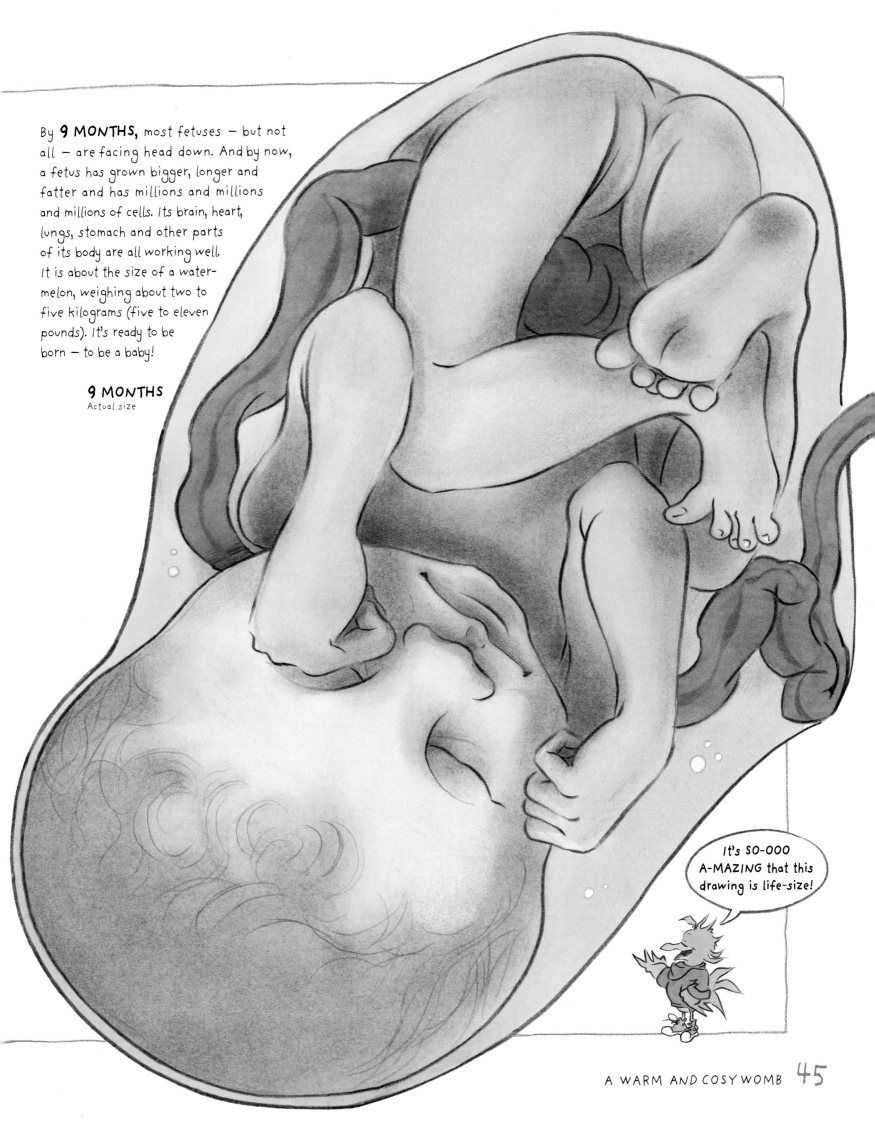

By **9 MONTHS,** most fetuses — but not all — are facing head down. And by now, a fetus has grown bigger, longer and fatter and has millions and millions and millions of cells. Its brain, heart, lungs, stomach and other parts of its body are all working well. It is about the size of a water-melon, weighing about two to five kilograms (five to eleven pounds). It's ready to be born — to be a baby!

9 MONTHS
Actual size

It's SO-OOO A-MAZING that this drawing is life-size!

FRESH FOOD! FRESH AIR!

Growing and Staying Healthy

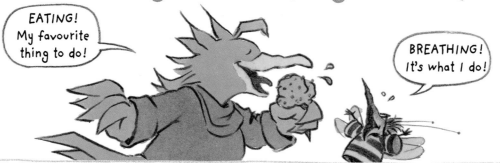

Inside the uterus, a sac filled with warm water surrounds the embryo – and then the fetus – and keeps it warm and safe as it grows. The sac is called the "amniotic sac". The fetus floats in the warm water. The warm water is called "amniotic fluid". The sac and the water protect the fetus from pokes and jolts and bumps.

Every so often, the fetus drinks some of the warm water it floats in. The water inside the uterus is perfectly healthy for a fetus to drink.

While the fetus is inside the uterus, it needs food and air, just like we all do, to grow and stay healthy. But a fetus cannot eat food the way we do or breathe air on its own.

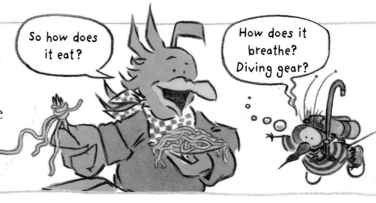

WARM AND SAFE IN THE UTERUS

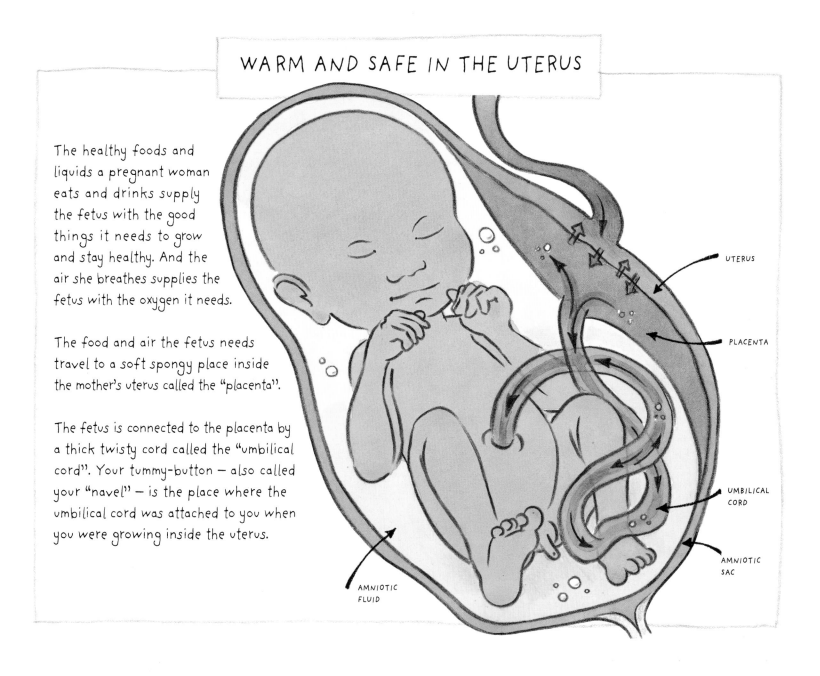

The healthy foods and liquids a pregnant woman eats and drinks supply the fetus with the good things it needs to grow and stay healthy. And the air she breathes supplies the fetus with the oxygen it needs.

The food and air the fetus needs travel to a soft spongy place inside the mother's uterus called the "placenta".

The fetus is connected to the placenta by a thick twisty cord called the "umbilical cord". Your tummy-button — also called your "navel" — is the place where the umbilical cord was attached to you when you were growing inside the uterus.

UTERUS

PLACENTA

UMBILICAL CORD

AMNIOTIC SAC

AMNIOTIC FLUID

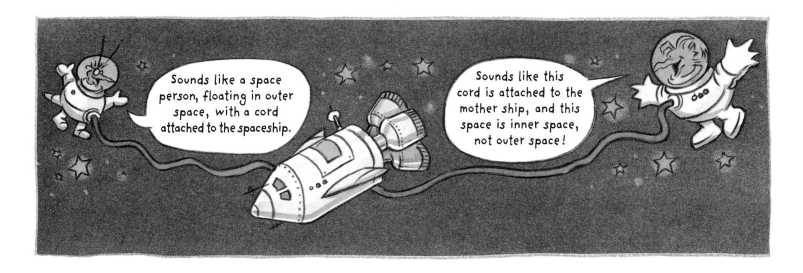

Sounds like a space person, floating in outer space, with a cord attached to the spaceship.

Sounds like this cord is attached to the mother ship, and this space is inner space, not outer space!

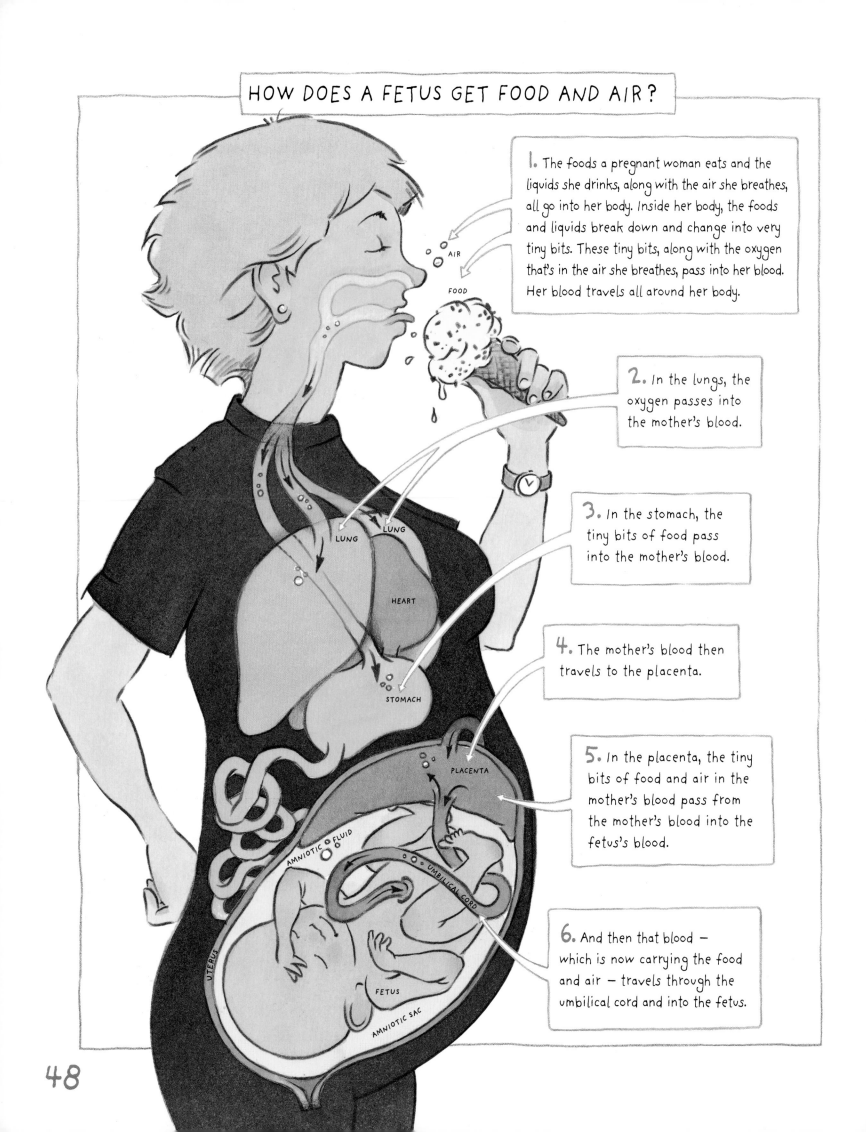

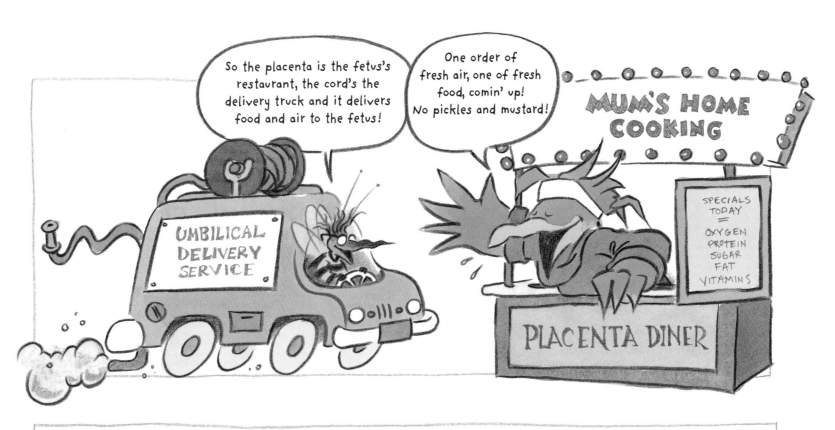

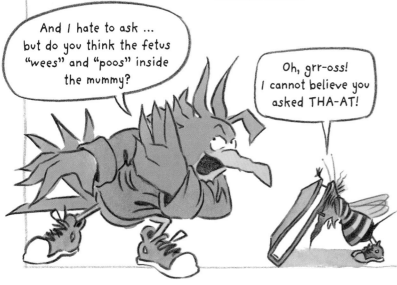

The bits of food and air the fetus does not need leave through the umbilical cord. Some bits of the food and air also leave the fetus's body in the small amount of urine – also called "wee" – it makes. The fetus's "wee" becomes part of the water in the uterus. Usually a fetus does not "poo" while it's in the uterus.

Sometimes unhealthy things can pass into a pregnant woman's blood and into the fetus – cigarette smoke and many kinds of drugs, including alcohol from wine, beer, or spirits. Most pregnant women are very careful about what they eat and drink and what medicines they take. They want to do everything possible to give birth to a healthy baby.

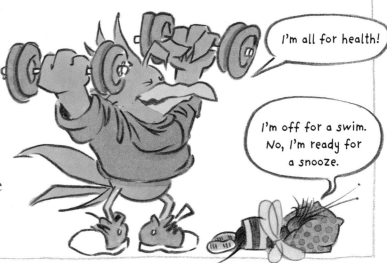

STRETCH! PUNCH! KICK! HICCUP! BURP!

The Growing Fetus

While a fetus is growing inside the uterus, it does a lot of things! It can make a fist and punch. It can kick its feet. It can even do somersaults. It can suck its thumb and fingers. And it can taste, swallow and blink and open its eyes. It can also stretch and sleep. And it can make noises – like hiccups and burps!

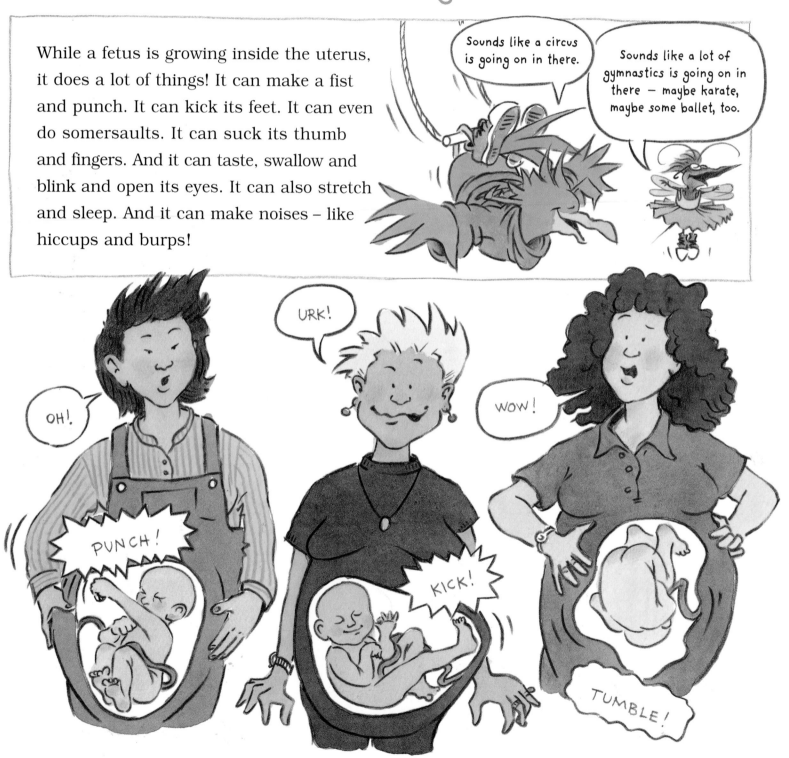

A fetus can also hear. It can hear the sound of its mother's voice, the sound of her stomach rumbling, the sound of her heart beating and of her blood pumping through her body.

It can hear noises like a doorbell ringing, or a piano being played, or a song being sung. You could do all of these things, too – when you were growing inside the uterus.

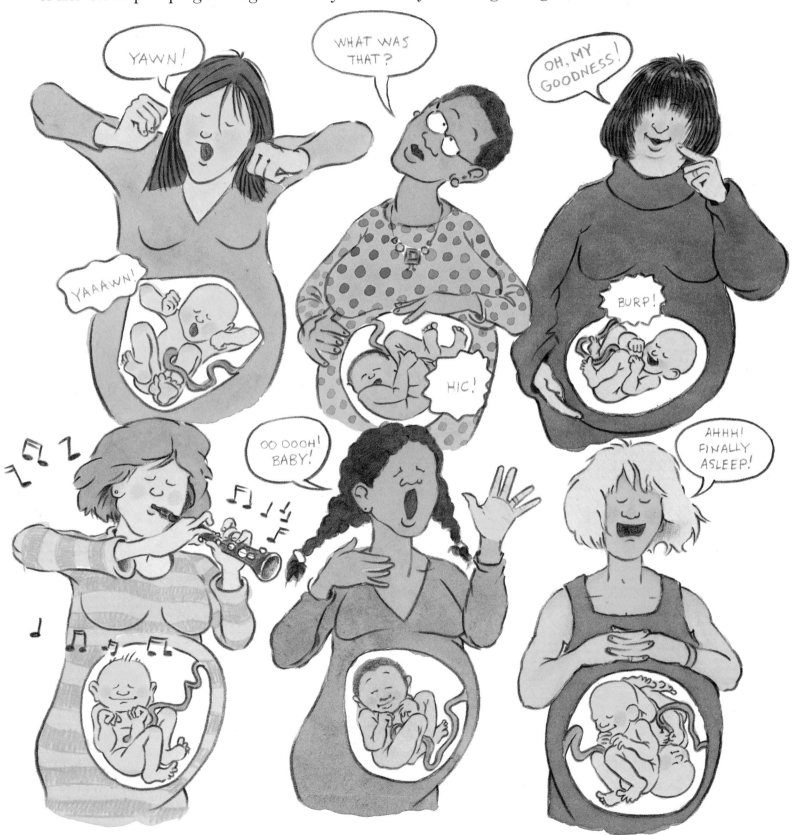

After a woman is about four or five months pregnant, at times she can feel the fetus moving. When a fetus hears a loud sound, or when a bright light or bright sunshine shines on the uterus, a fetus may move suddenly. A pregnant woman can feel when a fetus is moving a lot and when it is quiet and resting.

You might like to ask a woman who is pregnant – your mother or an aunt or a family friend or a friend's mother – if you can put your hand on her tummy. When a fetus has grown big enough, you may be able to see and feel the fetus move and stretch its arms and legs, or punch its fist, or kick its feet.

You may also be able to see the shape of the fetus's body, or elbow, or knee, or fist, or foot. And when the fetus moves, sometimes you can see that, too. Moving and stretching and kicking and punching don't hurt the mother at all – but she can feel it.

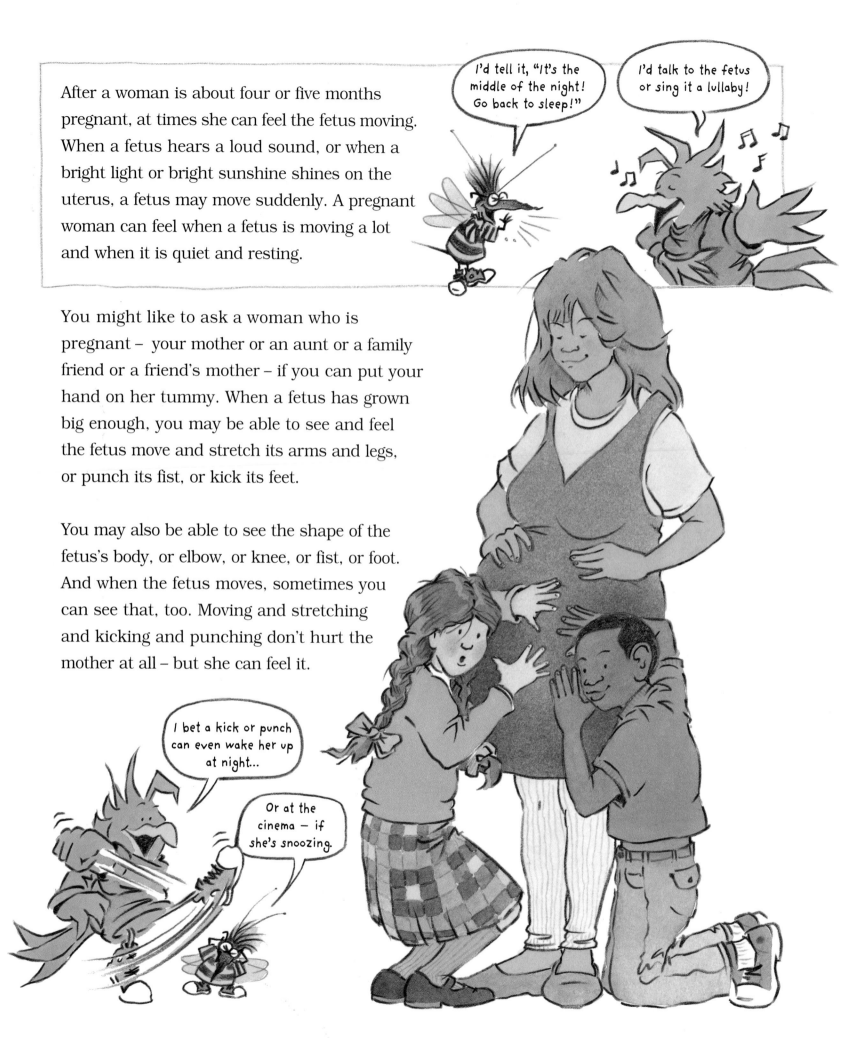

I'd tell it, "It's the middle of the night! Go back to sleep!"

I'd talk to the fetus or sing it a lullaby!

I bet a kick or punch can even wake her up at night...

Or at the cinema — if she's snoozing.

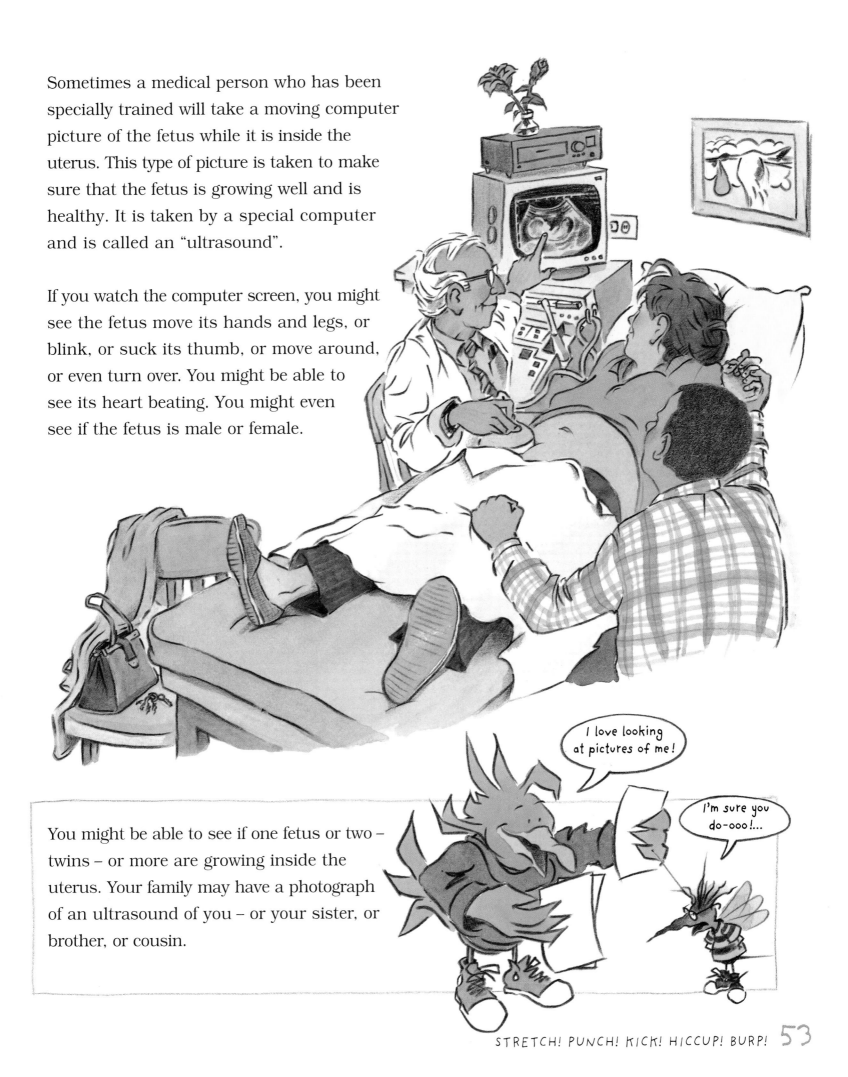

Sometimes a medical person who has been specially trained will take a moving computer picture of the fetus while it is inside the uterus. This type of picture is taken to make sure that the fetus is growing well and is healthy. It is taken by a special computer and is called an "ultrasound".

If you watch the computer screen, you might see the fetus move its hands and legs, or blink, or suck its thumb, or move around, or even turn over. You might be able to see its heart beating. You might even see if the fetus is male or female.

You might be able to see if one fetus or two – twins – or more are growing inside the uterus. Your family may have a photograph of an ultrasound of you – or your sister, or brother, or cousin.

I love looking at pictures of me!

I'm sure you do-ooo!...

TWINS AND MORE!
Twins, Triplets, Quadruplets, Quintuplets

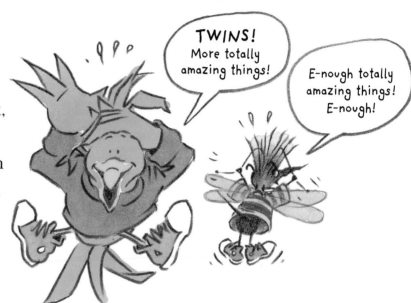

Most of the time when a sperm and egg meet, the beginning cells of only one baby start to grow. But another amazing thing can happen the moment an egg and sperm meet. Although it does not happen often, the beginning cells of two babies – twins – can start to grow.

HOW DO TWINS BEGIN?

Identical Twins

If an egg that has been fertilized by a sperm splits into two while it is in the Fallopian tube, the beginning cells of two babies — identical twins — can start to grow in the uterus.

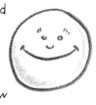 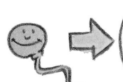 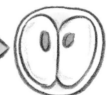 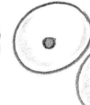

| 1 egg | + | 1 sperm | join and split in 2 | = | the beginning cells of identical twins |

Fraternal Twins

Twins can also begin if two eggs happen to be in the Fallopian tube. If those two eggs join with two sperm, the beginning cells of two babies — fraternal twins — can start to grow in the uterus.

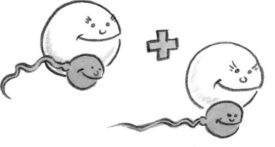 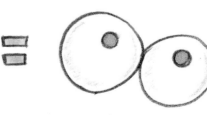

1 egg and 1 sperm   +   1 egg and 1 sperm   =   the beginning cells of fraternal twins

Identical Twins

Identical means "the same". Identical twins look almost exactly alike and are always the same sex. When identical twins are born, they are always either two girls or two boys.

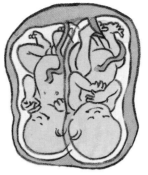

2 GIRLS   OR   2 BOYS

Fraternal Twins

Fraternal twins do not look exactly alike. When fraternal twins are born, they are either a boy and a girl, two boys, or two girls.

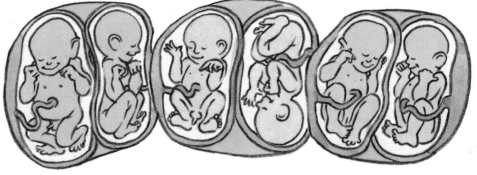

A BOY AND A GIRL   OR   2 BOYS   OR   2 GIRLS

Triplets

If three eggs and three sperm join together in the Fallopian tube, or if a fertilized egg splits into three, the beginning cells of three babies — triplets — can start to grow in the uterus.

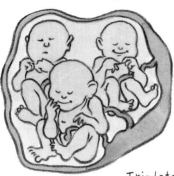

Quadruplets

Sometimes, the beginning cells of four babies — quadruplets — can start to grow in the uterus.

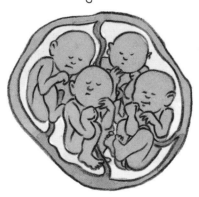

Quintuplets

Sometimes, the beginning cells of five babies — quintuplets — can start to grow in the uterus.

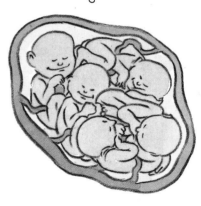

Triplets, quadruplets, and quintuplets — like twins — can be identical or fraternal. Or they can be a mixture of both.

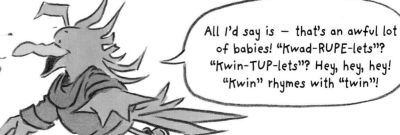

TRI means "three", QUAD means "four", and QUIN means "five" — in Latin. What I bet you can say is "TRIP-lets". But can you say "QUAD-rup-lets"? Or "QUIN-tup-lets"?

All I'd say is — that's an awful lot of babies! "Kwad-RUPE-lets"? "Kwin-TUP-lets"? Hey, hey, hey! "Kwin" rhymes with "twin"!

COME OUT, COME OUT, WHEREVER YOU ARE!

Birth

After nine months inside the uterus, the fetus has grown big enough and strong enough and is ready to be born. Being born can take a long time – sometimes more than a day. Or it can take just a few hours.

How does the baby know when to come out?

Someone must shout, "Come out, come out, wherever you are!"

Most babies are born in hospitals. Some babies are born at home. People who are specially trained – a midwife or doctor – help the mother while her baby is being born. Fathers, and sometimes other family members and friends, often help, too.

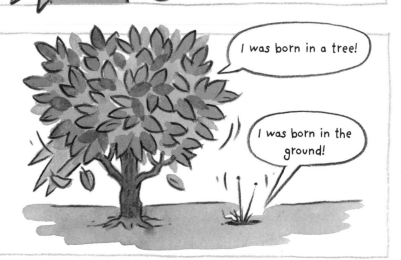

I was born in a tree!

I was born in the ground!

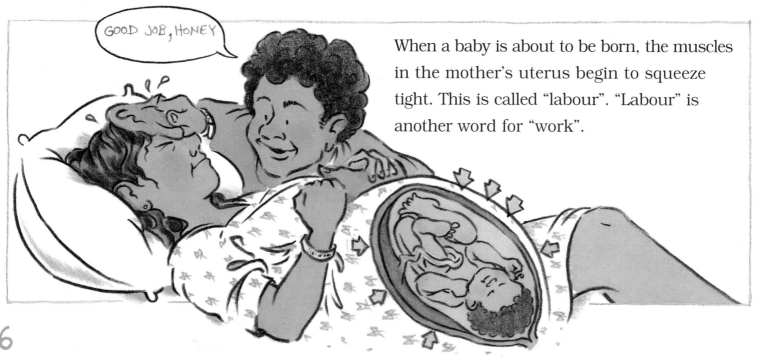

GOOD JOB, HONEY

When a baby is about to be born, the muscles in the mother's uterus begin to squeeze tight. This is called "labour". "Labour" is another word for "work".

A mother's muscles work very hard to push and squeeze the baby out of the uterus and into the vagina. Then the mother's muscles push and squeeze the baby's body through the vagina.

The vagina stretches wide as the baby's soft, wet and slippery body travels through it. It's a tight squeeze, but finally the baby slides out – and is born!

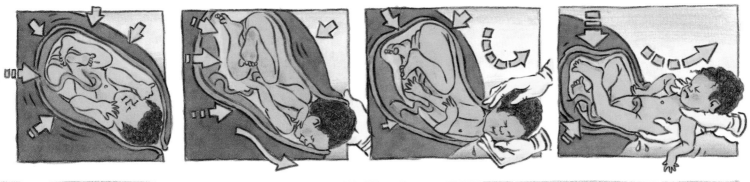

The moment of birth is so exciting! The doctor or midwife, or sometimes the baby's father, gently holds the baby as it comes out. That's when most babies let out their first cry. And that's when someone almost always shouts out, "It's a girl!" or "It's a boy!"

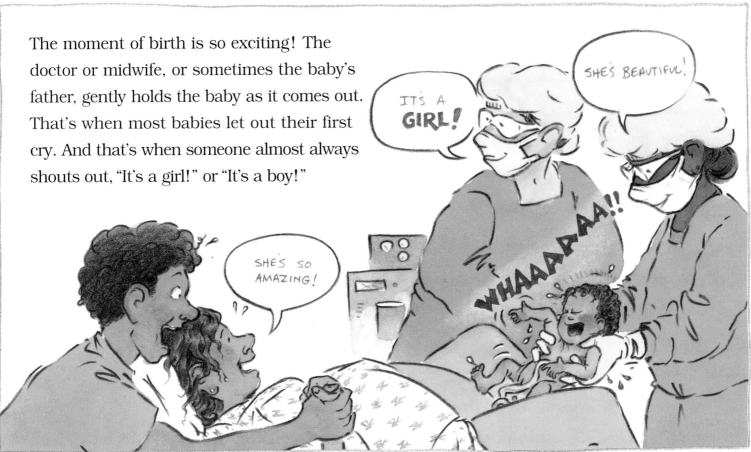

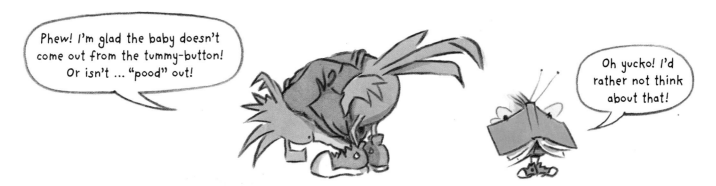

Whether it is soft or loud, a baby's first cry fills up its lungs with fresh air. This is how a baby takes its first breath and starts breathing on its own.

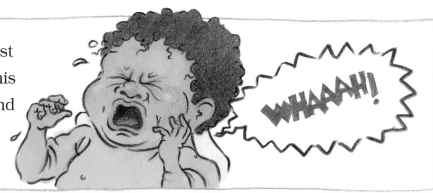

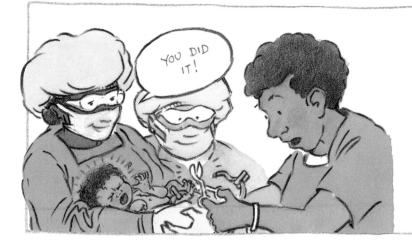

Minutes later, the doctor – or sometimes a midwife or the baby's father – cuts the cord. This is the cord that connected the baby to its mother and gave it food and air. The cord is cut because the mother no longer needs to eat and breathe for the baby. The cutting does not hurt the baby or the mother.

As soon as the cord is cut – or sometimes even before – the baby's parents are usually able to hold, cuddle, kiss, and hug their new baby. It feels so wonderful when a parent can finally hold and look at the new baby.

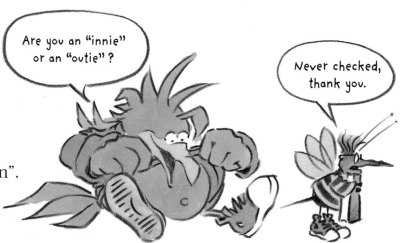

The tiny piece of cord that is left on the baby's body dries up and falls off, after a week or so. The place where the cord was attached becomes a person's navel. It often looks like a button, and that's probably why many people call the navel a "tummy-button".

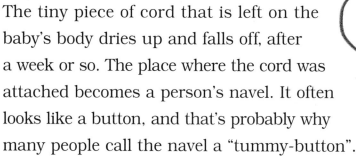

A few minutes later, the placenta and amniotic sac pass out of the mother's body through her vagina. The placenta is no longer needed to help the baby eat and breathe. The sac is no longer needed to hold and protect the baby.

I can breathe and eat on my own.

Speaking of eating — I'm hungry!

PIZZA

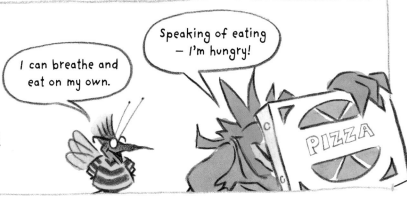

Most babies are born head first. Some are born bottom first. And most are born through the vagina. But if a baby is too big, or is in a difficult position in the uterus – like sideways – the doctor makes a cut through the mother's skin and into her uterus. The mother is given some medicine before the cut is made, so she won't feel pain. After the cut is made, the baby is lifted out – and is born!

Then the umbilical cord is cut. The placenta and amniotic sac are lifted out and the cut in the mother's skin and uterus is sewn with a special thread. This cut heals in a few weeks' time. When a baby is born this way, it is called a "cesarean birth" or a "c-section". A cesarean birth is another perfectly normal and healthy way to be born.

IT'S A BOY!

WHAAAAA!!

HE'S SO AMAZING!

HE'S BEAUTIFUL!

It says here:
"The name 'cesarean' comes from the name of the great Roman leader Julius Caesar. Historians believe that Caesar may have been born this way in ancient Rome around 100 B.C. – more than 2,000 years ago."
Now THAT is interesting!

If it was good enough for Caesar, it's good enough for me.

Some babies are born before they have spent a whole nine months in the uterus. Babies who are born early are called "premature" babies or "prems". Prems often have to stay in the hospital for some extra time until they learn to suck well. This helps them eat well. They also need to stay until they have gained enough weight to keep their bodies warm enough.

My feathers keep me warm!

I flutter my wings and fly around a lot. That keeps me warm!

While they are in the hospital, prems usually sleep in a special cot called an "incubator". The incubator keeps the baby warm and provides fresh air for the baby to breathe as it continues to grow.

A prem's parent or parents spend lots of time in the hospital getting to know their baby. They can touch, hold, kiss, talk to, sing to and feed their baby.

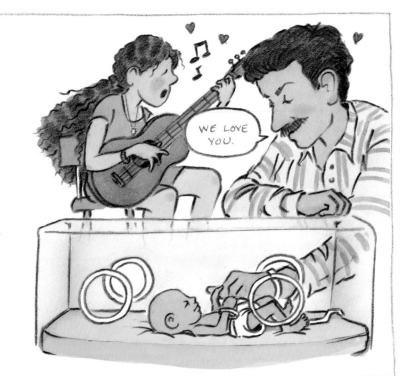

WE LOVE YOU.

When the baby grows bigger and stronger, its parents or parent can take their baby home.

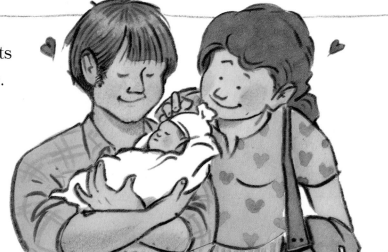

New babies need to be fed. Milk is the only food they need until they are older. After a baby is born, its mother's breasts begin to make milk. When a baby sucks and drinks milk from its mother's breasts, the mother's breasts make more milk. Breast milk contains all the vitamins, sugars, fats, salt, and other things a young baby needs to grow and stay healthy. Sometimes babies are fed breast milk from a bottle.

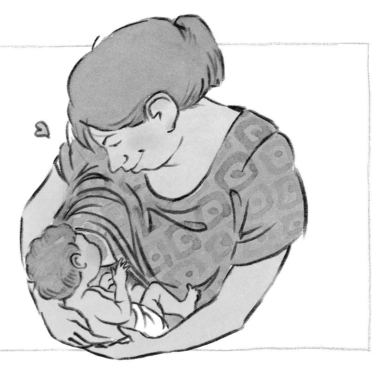

Some babies are fed milk – called "formula" – from a bottle. This milk is different from breast milk. Formula is made from cow's milk or soya milk, which is made from the bean of the soyabean plant. Vitamins, sugars, fats, salt and other things are added to help a young baby grow and stay healthy. Babies suck and drink formula from a rubber teat that's attached to a bottle.

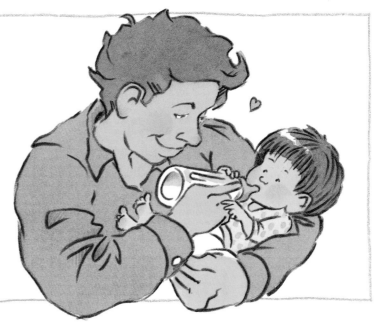

When babies are a few months old, they can start to eat other foods. And by their first birthday, most babies can drink cow's milk – just like most older children and grown-ups do.

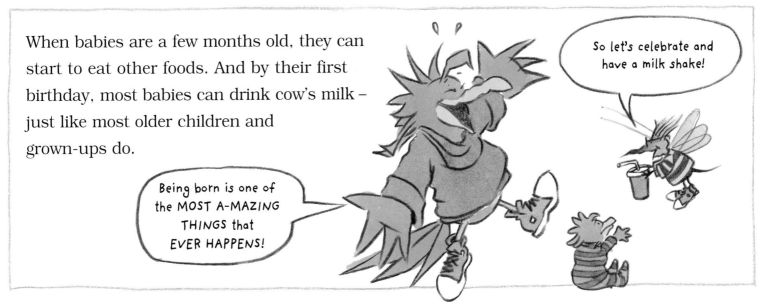

So let's celebrate and have a milk shake!

Being born is one of the MOST A-MAZING THINGS that EVER HAPPENS!

WHAT MAKES YOU-YOU!
Chromosomes and Genes – And Other Things, Too!

You may wonder how you happened to be born a boy or a girl, or with curly hair instead of straight hair. These things are decided the moment a sperm cell and an egg cell join together – long before a baby is born.

> Back to egg and sperm again?

> Yep! That's when what makes you YOU starts!

Inside every egg and sperm are chromosomes. Chromosomes look like tiny threads and are so small they can be seen only under a microscope. All sperm have an X or a Y chromosome. All eggs have an X chromosome.

If a sperm with a Y chromosome joins with an egg, a male baby – a boy – will be born. If a sperm with an X chromosome joins with an egg, a female baby – a girl – will be born. That's how it was decided what gender or sex you are – female or male.

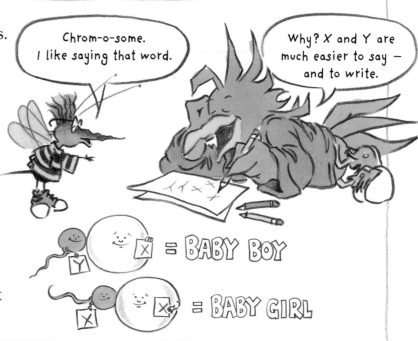

> Chrom-o-some. I like saying that word.

> Why? X and Y are much easier to say – and to write.

= BABY BOY

= BABY GIRL

Strung along our chromosomes – like beads on a necklace – are tiny, tiny parts called "genes". Genes contain thousands of pieces of information about a person – such as whether a person has brown or blue eyes, or small or large hands. Your genes were passed on to you from your parents when the sperm and the egg that made you joined together.

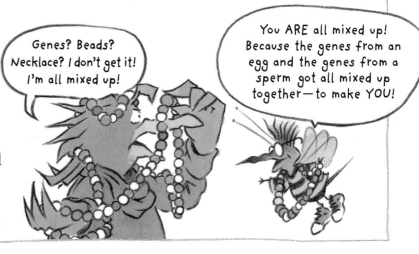

> Genes? Beads? Necklace? I don't get it! I'm all mixed up!

> You ARE all mixed up! Because the genes from an egg and the genes from a sperm got all mixed up together—to make YOU!

The colour of your eyes and hair and skin, the size of your feet, the shape of your ears, the shape of your body, how short or tall you are – and thousands of other things about you – were all passed on to you from your parents' genes. If you were adopted, your genes were passed on to you by the woman and man – called your "birth parents" – whose egg and sperm joined to make you.

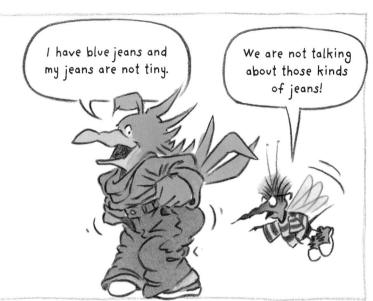

But you are not an exact copy of either parent whose sperm and egg joined together to make you. That's because you received a mixture of genes from both of them, and from their parents and grandparents, and from their ancestors. That's why if you have a brother or sister, you can look somewhat different – or very different – from each other. That's why you may look a lot like your parents – or hardly at all like your parents.

Who you are is not decided by genes and chromosomes alone. All the people you grow up with, all the things you do, all that happens to you – along with all the genes that mixed together to make you – are what make you different from any other person. That's why no person in the world is exactly like you – even if you are an identical twin.

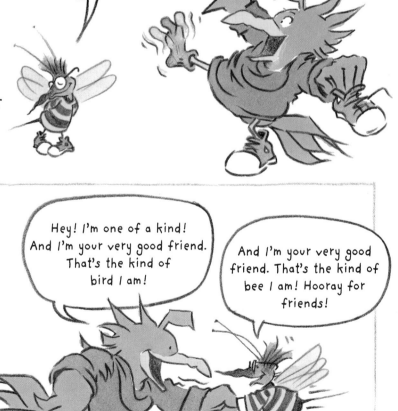

BECOMING A FAMILY
By Birth — By Adoption

Every family is different. Almost all babies and children grow up in families and are taken care of by their families. Babies and children grow up in all sorts of families.

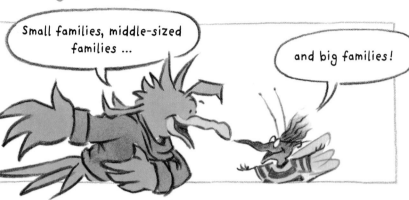

Small families, middle-sized families ...

and big families!

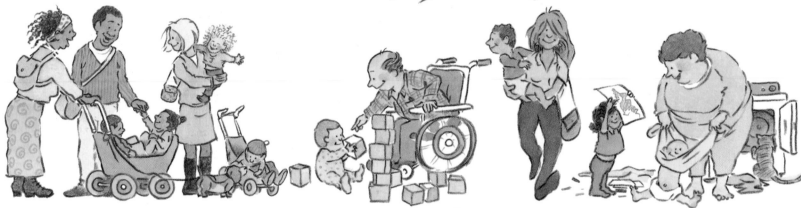

There are children whose parents are married, and children whose parents live together and are not married. There are children whose parents are divorced and live apart, and children whose parents live apart but are not divorced.

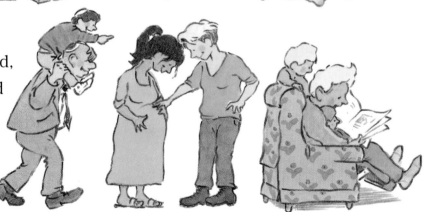

There are children who grow up with their birth parents, and children whose parent or parents have adopted them. There are children who grow up with one parent. There are children who live with one parent part of the time and with their other parent the rest of the time.

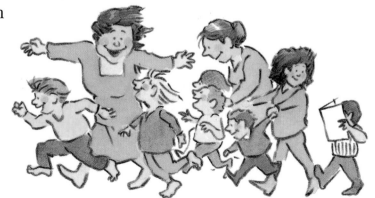

There are children whose parent or parents are gay men, and children whose parent or parents are lesbian women. There are children who live with a parent and a stepparent, or who live with an aunt, an uncle, a grandmother, a grandfather, or other relatives. Sometimes children live with a foster parent or parents while their own parent or parents or a social worker works out who would be the best person to take loving and good care of them.

Hey! All kinds of families!

Hey! All kinds of children!

Parents, grandparents, cousins, uncles, and aunts are all part of a person's family. And for many people, good friends are part of their families, too. Most children are loved and taken care of by family members and family friends.

Most babies are born into their family. Some babies are adopted into their family. But the beginning cell of every baby starts when a woman's egg and a man's sperm join and become one cell. This united egg-and-sperm cell divides again and again and travels to the woman's uterus – where it grows until a baby is born. That woman and that man are your parents unless you were adopted.

If you were adopted, the woman whose egg helped to make you is called your "birth mother" or "biological mother". And the man whose sperm helped to make you is called your "birth father" or "biological father".

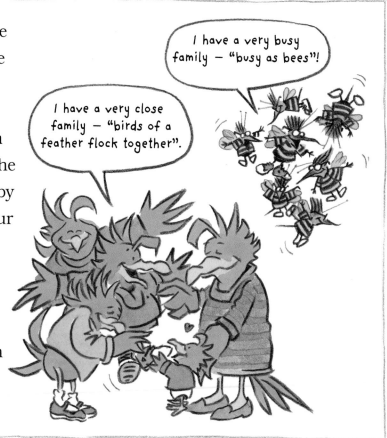

There are times when a birth mother or birth father or birth parents cannot take care of their baby or child. When this happens, they make a plan for their baby or child to be adopted – to become a member of another family and be cared for and loved by that family.

Some people choose to adopt because they are not able to give birth to a child. Other people who can give or have given birth to a baby also choose to adopt.

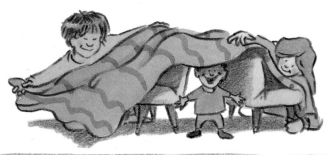

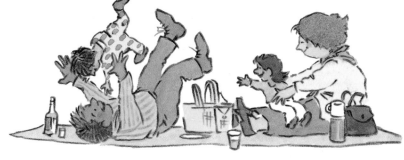

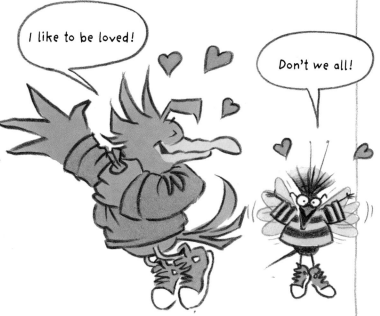

When a parent or parents adopt a child, that means they will love and raise that baby or child as their own child. In the UK, when a child is adopted, the new adoptive parent or parents and the child must go to court, so that a judge can approve the adoption. And the adoptive parent or parents sign a paper and agree in front of the judge to care for, raise and protect the child they have chosen to adopt.

In the Republic of Ireland, the new adoptive parent or parents and the child must go to an Adoption Board of up to nine people so that the Board can approve the adoption. In Australia, usually the new adoptive parent or parents and the child must go to court or to a judge's office, so that a judge can approve the adoption. In all three countries, when a parent or parents who are citizens living in their country adopt a child, that child can become a citizen of the adoptive parent's or parents' country.

When a baby or child is adopted, its parent or parents often have a party or ceremony and invite family members to meet and celebrate their new baby or child. Choosing to adopt a baby or child is another way for a grown-up to become a parent and for a baby or child to be cared for and loved.

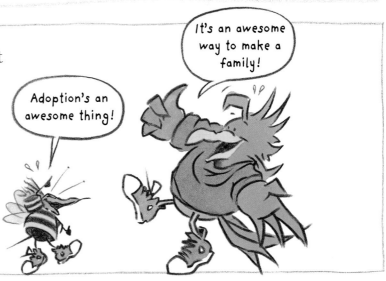

Adoption's an awesome thing!

It's an awesome way to make a family!

KEEPING SAFE
"OK Touches"—"Not OK Touches"

Every family's job is to love, take care of, and keep their babies and children safe. One very important thing to know about staying safe is that your body belongs to you.

The female parts of girls' and women's bodies and the male parts of boys' and men's bodies are often called "private parts". The private parts of a person's body are the parts that are usually covered by underpants or by a swimsuit or trunks.

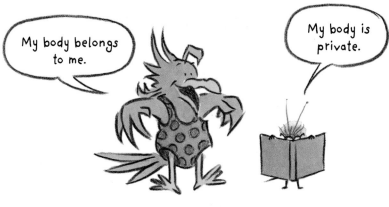

My body belongs to me.

My body is private.

When your parent takes you to the doctor, the reason your doctor may have to look at and touch the private parts of your body is to make sure every part of your body is healthy.

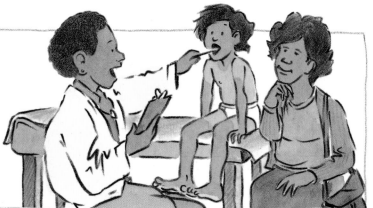

If your private parts ever feel uncomfortable or hurt, it's important to tell a parent, or another adult you know well and trust. Then that person can take you to the doctor. Always tell the doctor if any part of your body hurts, or has been hurt, or feels uncomfortable.

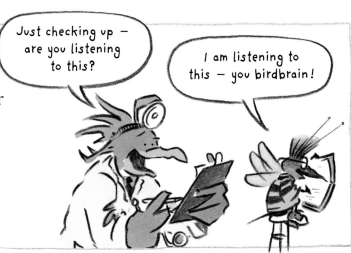

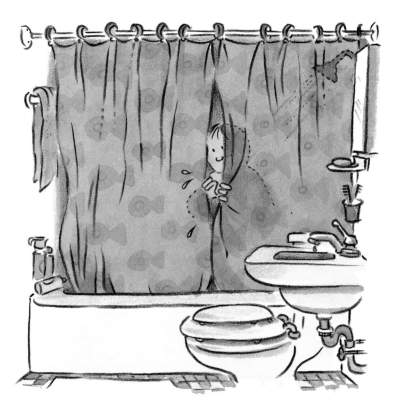

It's perfectly normal to be curious about your own body – how it looks, feels, and works. It's also perfectly normal to want some private time for yourself and to have some privacy when you are getting dressed or having a bath or a shower.

Touching or rubbing the private parts of your own body because it feels good is called "masturbation". Some people also call masturbation "playing with yourself". Many people masturbate. Many don't.

Every family has its own thoughts and feelings about masturbation. Your family may feel differently from your friend's or cousin's or neighbour's family about whether it's OK, or not OK, to masturbate. Some people and some religions think it's wrong to masturbate. But most doctors agree that masturbation is perfectly healthy and perfectly normal and cannot hurt you or your body.

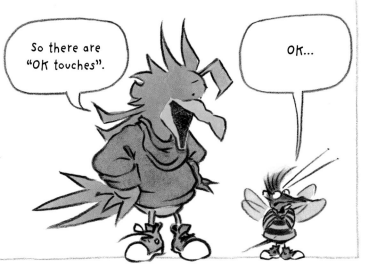

But if any person touches any part of your body and you do not want them to, say "STOP!" or "NO!" or "DON'T!" It is your right to say that – even if the person is someone in your family or someone you know, even if the person is bigger, older, or stronger than you are.

You may have heard the words "sexual abuse". Sexual abuse happens when someone touches the private parts of a person's body and does NOT have the right to do that.

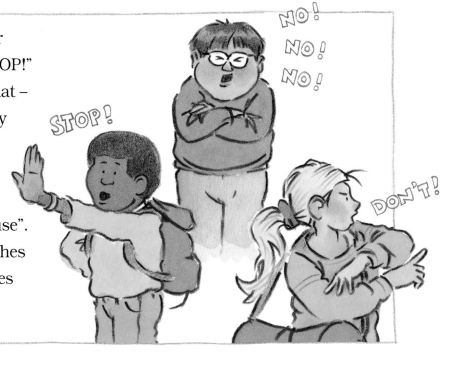

Sexual abuse is always wrong, and most adults know that it is wrong. Sexual abuse can hurt. Or it can feel gentle. This can be very confusing because it's almost impossible to understand how something so wrong can feel gentle.

If sexual abuse ever happens to you – it is NEVER your fault. And do NOT keep it a secret even if someone tells you to keep it a secret. There are some secrets that are OK to keep, but sexual abuse is not one of them. You must make sure that you tell another person straight away – someone in your family, or your teacher, or doctor, or nurse, or school nurse, or clergy member, or someone you know very well and trust.

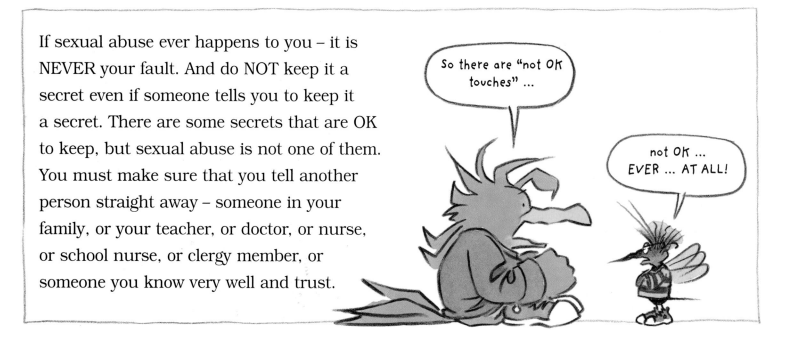

Most of the time, the person you tell will do all he or she can to stop the abuse from happening again. But if the first person you tell doesn't listen or believe you, tell a second person. Talk about it until you find someone who does listen and believes you. He or she will try to keep you safe and protect you from the person who tried to touch you or did touch you. Most adults *do* care about children and want to keep them safe.

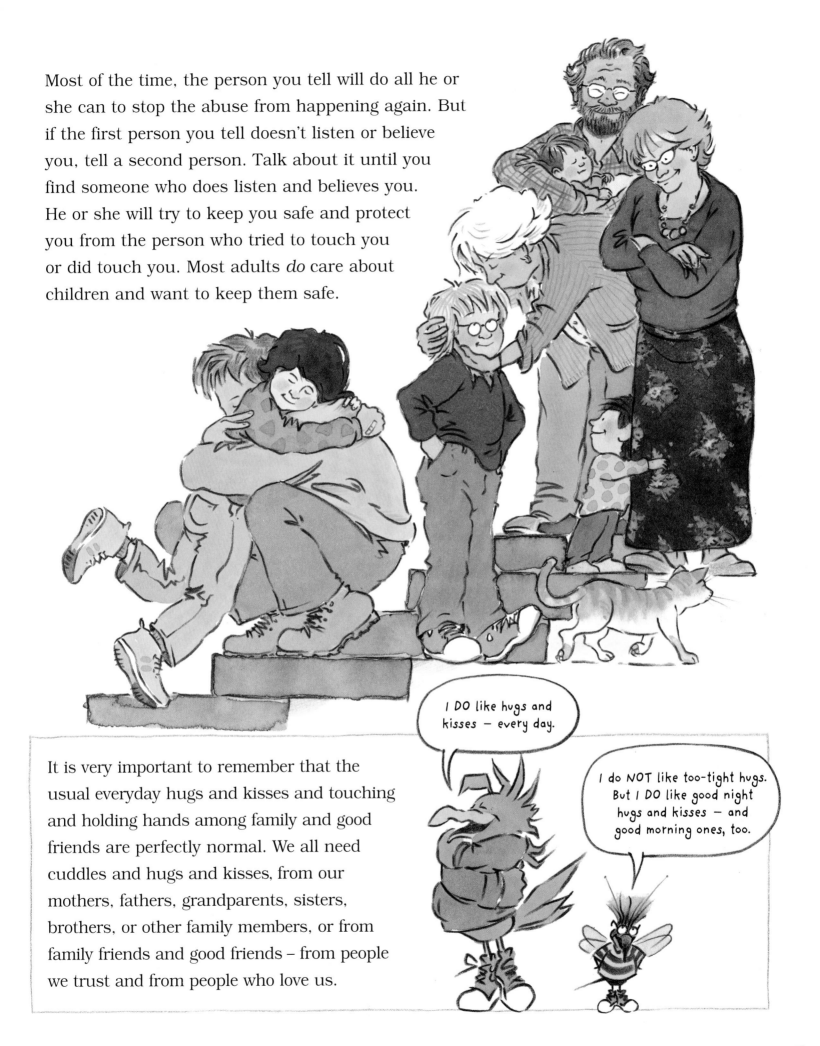

I DO like hugs and kisses — every day.

I do NOT like too-tight hugs. But I DO like good night hugs and kisses — and good morning ones, too.

It is very important to remember that the usual everyday hugs and kisses and touching and holding hands among family and good friends are perfectly normal. We all need cuddles and hugs and kisses, from our mothers, fathers, grandparents, sisters, brothers, or other family members, or from family friends and good friends – from people we trust and from people who love us.

TALKING ABOUT IT
HIV and AIDS

The chances are you know something about HIV and AIDS. You may even have heard that HIV can have something to do with sex – or with drugs and needles. Wanting to know about HIV and AIDS is perfectly normal. And knowing about them can help to keep people safe from getting HIV and AIDS.

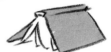

> Hearing about HIV and AIDS is scary...

> Talking about it is scary, too...

KNOWING ABOUT HIV AND AIDS

HIV is the virus – the germ – that causes AIDS. A virus is a germ that can cause a person to become sick. Most germs – like colds and flu – usually cause people to become sick for only a short time and then they get better. A person who has HIV may stay well and feel healthy for many years. But when a person who has HIV develops AIDS, he or she may become very sick and may not get better.

It is very sad that so many people who have had AIDS have died. But scientists have discovered some medicines that are helping more and more people who have HIV to feel better and live longer. And scientists are working day and night trying to find even better ways to keep people safe from getting HIV and to help people who have HIV. Scientists have also discovered ways people CANNOT get HIV and CAN get HIV.

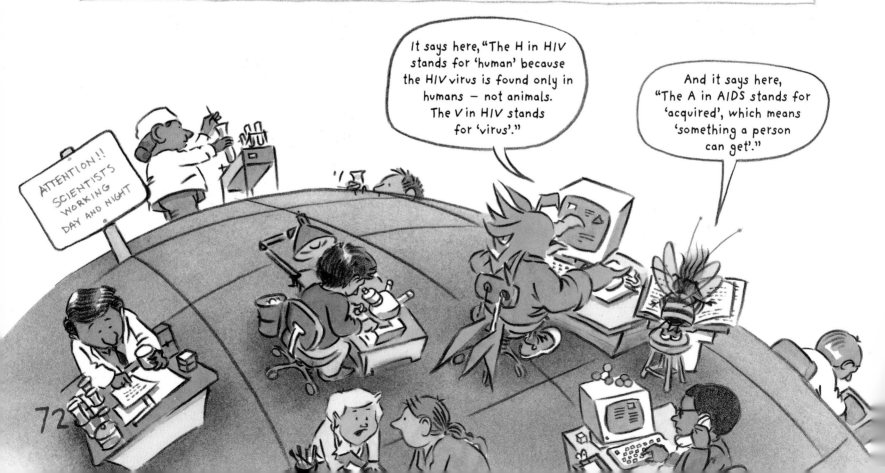

> It says here, "The H in HIV stands for 'human' because the HIV virus is found only in humans – not animals. The V in HIV stands for 'virus'."

> And it says here, "The A in AIDS stands for 'acquired', which means 'something a person can get'."

72

WAYS A PERSON **CANNOT** GET HIV

• A person CANNOT get HIV from going to school or work with a person who has HIV, from playing with a person who has HIV, from hugging a person who has HIV, or from giving a high-five or a kiss hello or good-bye to someone who has HIV.

• A person CANNOT get HIV from a cough or a sneeze, or an insect bite, or from sitting on the same toilet seat that someone with HIV has sat on, or from swimming in the same pool with someone who has HIV.

• A person CANNOT get HIV from a brand-new, clean and germfree needle that a doctor or nurse uses to give injections, or from a brand-new, clean, and germfree needle that is used to pierce ears for earrings.

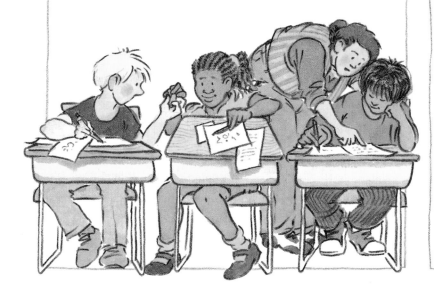

WAYS A PERSON **CAN** GET HIV

• A person CAN get HIV from having sexual intercourse with a person who has HIV. Other infections can also be passed from one person to another during sexual intercourse. When people have sexual intercourse, wearing a condom can help keep a person safe from getting HIV or passing HIV – or some other infections – from one person to another.

• A person CAN get HIV from blood in or on drug, tattoo or ear-piercing needles that have been used by someone who has HIV. That's because people with HIV have the virus in their blood. Other infections can also be passed from one person to another by sharing needles.

• If a pregnant woman has HIV, sometimes the virus CAN be passed on to her fetus – and her baby COULD be born with HIV. A pregnant woman who has HIV can take a medicine that can help to keep her baby from being born with HIV. And some babies – but not all – CAN get HIV from their mother's breast milk if the mother has HIV.

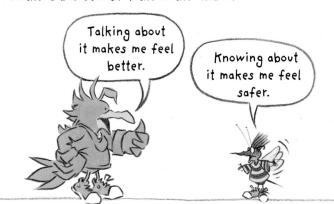

Talking about it makes me feel better.

Knowing about it makes me feel safer.

People who have HIV, and babies and children who are born with HIV, often stay well and feel healthy for many years. It's important to treat a person who has been infected with HIV, or who has AIDS, as you would treat any friend. Give a hug, a high-five, or a kiss hello to that person. Play with, hang out with, go to a film with, or ride bikes with that person – and do the many things you like to do with a good friend.

GURGLES AND DROOLS
Feelings about Babies – Fun with Babies

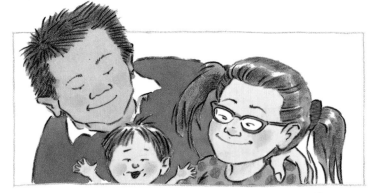

No matter how or when you arrived – or whether you are an only child, the youngest child, a middle child, or the oldest child in your family – you will always have a very special place in your family.

If you are an older brother or sister and there is a new baby in your family, you may have a lot of feelings about the new baby. At times, you may feel happy and even excited.

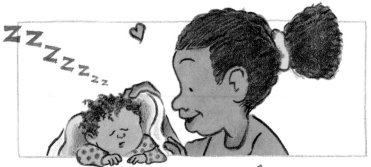

At other times, you may feel disappointed that the new baby is so small and can't do the kinds of things you can do – like reading books, playing football, eating spaghetti, flying a kite, baking biscuits, or singing a song.

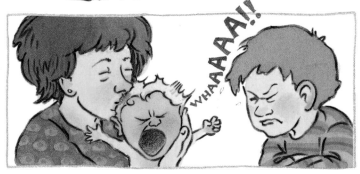

Sometimes, you may feel angry with your mother or father for having a new baby, or feel left out or sad. You may wish that your mother or father would be with you instead of the new baby. You may even feel angry with the new baby. And at times, you may not feel like helping out with or taking care of the new baby.

I really don't like helping out with those nappies!

I really don't like it when a baby cries.

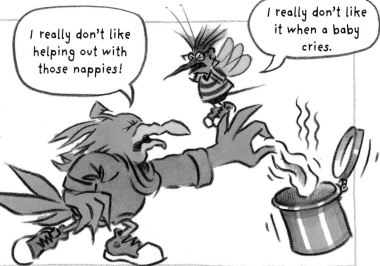

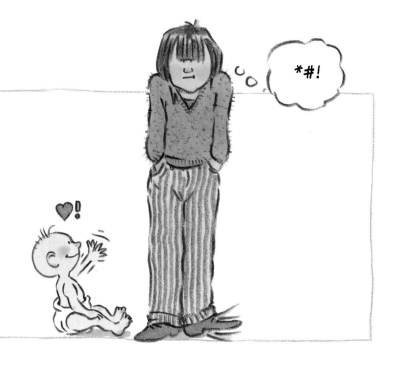

Having any of those feelings about a baby brother or sister, or about a baby cousin, or a friend's baby sister or brother, is perfectly normal. Most children have these kinds of feelings. But the truth is – babies love to be with older children. They learn so much by being with older children like you and watching what you do.

WAYS TO HAVE FUN WITH A BABY

Try whispering, or talking, or even singing to a baby. Try making a silly face. The chances are the baby will love that. Babies love to look at faces most of all. But don't get too close to the baby's face. Babies can get scared and may cry if you do.

When a baby gets tired or bored, the baby will tell you — by turning his or her head away, or crying, or falling asleep. Babies gurgle and drool a lot when you play and talk with them. That means they are having a good time with you. Babies like to have fun.

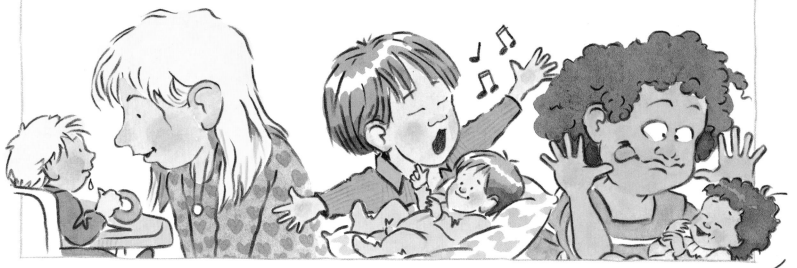

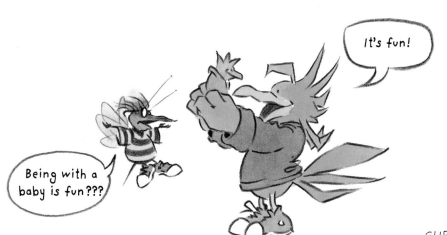

LET'S CELEBRATE!

Happy Birth Day! Happy Adoption Day!

All around the world, the arrival or adoption of a baby or child is usually one of the most exciting and amazing events ever!

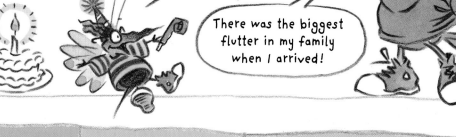

In the United States, many families hang brightly coloured balloons or a banner with the words "It's a GIRL!" or "It's a BOY!" outside their home. Some families put pink or blue ribbons on their front door.

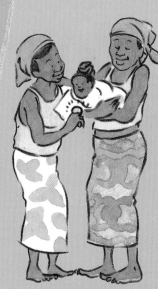

In the highlands of Kenya where the Gusii people live, mothers who have a new baby walk to a place where paths cross. When people walk by, they wish the baby well and give the mother a coin to bring the baby good luck and good health.

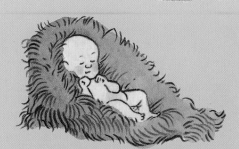

In Russia, when a new baby arrives home, the baby is laid on a fur to bring the baby good luck, good health and wealth.

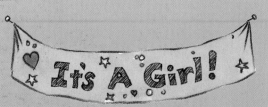

In many countries, including the UK, Australia and the Republic of Ireland, families send out cards or letters — often with a photograph — or put a few lines in the newspaper to announce the arrival of a new baby or child.

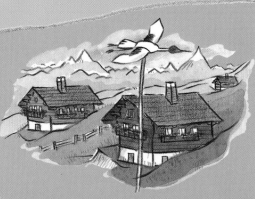

In the mountains of Switzerland, families hang a toy stork and other baby toys on a pole outside the house to tell everyone that a new baby has arrived.

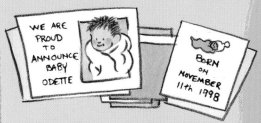

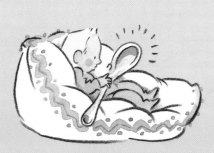

In Finland, a baby is given a piece of silver — often a spoon — when the baby is one month old. Every year, for the next twelve years, the child is given another piece of silver to celebrate its childhood.

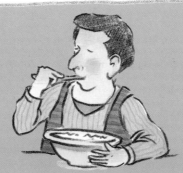

In Lebanon, a special rice pudding with nuts is made by someone in the new baby's family. Everyone who visits the baby eats a spoonful of the pudding to wish the baby good health.

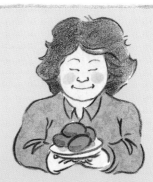

In parts of China, a new baby's parent or parents give eggs that have been dyed red to other family members and friends to celebrate the baby's arrival. The colour red stands for happiness, celebration and good luck.

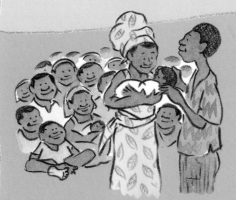

In Nigeria, eight days after a baby is born, every person who knows the baby's family comes to a ceremony at which the mother and father name the baby.

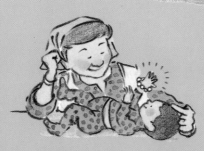

In Armenia, soon after a baby is home, the baby is given a bracelet with beads and blue stones that look like eyes to protect the baby from evil and harm.

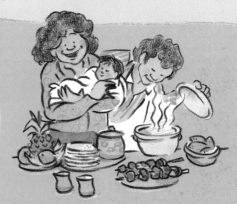

In parts of Costa Rica, a baby's family and friends bring a meal to the baby's home, so that the parents do not have to cook any meals for several days.

All around the world, families and friends celebrate the arrival of a baby or child in different ways. But one thing is the same for almost every family: families love to celebrate because they are so happy and so excited that a baby or child has become part of their family.

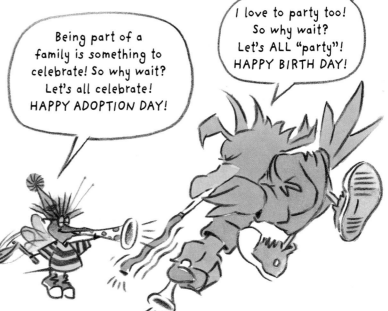

Being part of a family is something to celebrate! So why wait? Let's all celebrate! HAPPY ADOPTION DAY!

I love to party too! So why wait? Let's ALL "party"! HAPPY BIRTH DAY!

IT'S SO AMAZING!
Still Talking!

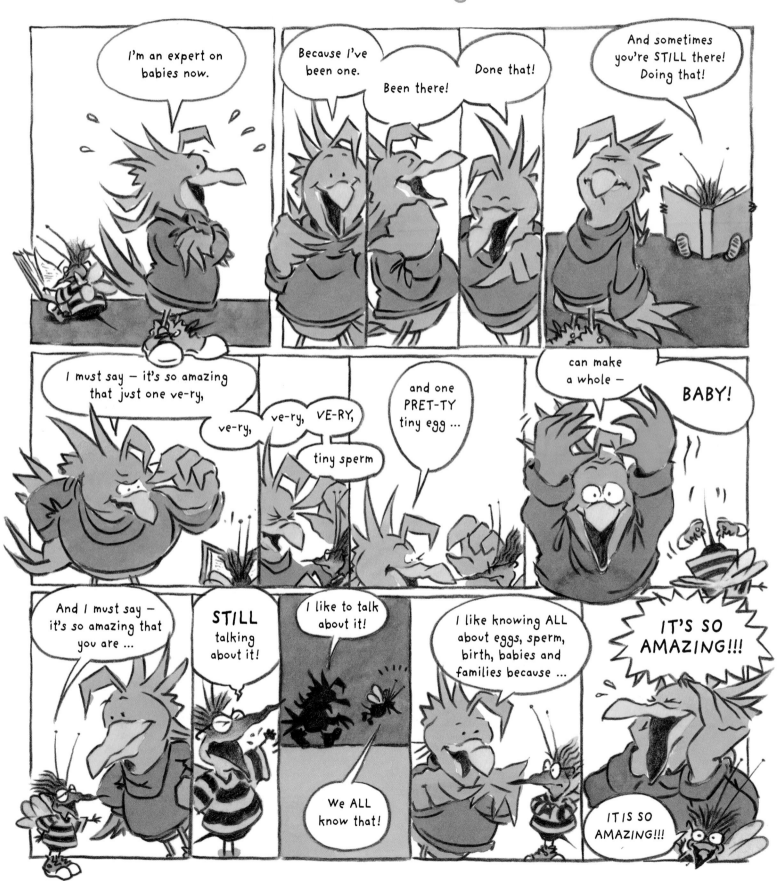

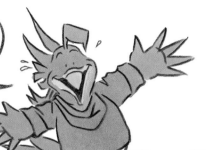

Thank you to ALL these people who ALL helped with this book!

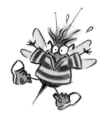

And ALL these people care about children. So thank you ALL!

REVEREND JORY AGATE, Unitarian Universalist Association, Boston, Massachusetts

TINA ALU, sexuality education coordinator, Cambridge Family Planning, Cambridge, Massachusetts

MARIE BARATTA, administrator, Cambridge, Massachusetts

ELIZABETH BARTHOLET, J.D., professor, Harvard Law School, Cambridge, Massachusetts

FRAN BASCHE, sexuality education trainer, Watertown, Massachusetts

TONI BELFIELD, Director of Information, fpa (Family Planning Association), London, England

EMILY BERKMAN, M.D., pediatrician, New York, New York

MERTON BERNFIELD, M.D., professor of pediatrics, director, Joint Program in Neonatology, Harvard Medical School, Children's Hospital, Boston, Massachusetts

SARAH BIRSS, M.D., pediatrician/child psychiatrist, Cambridge, Massachusetts

ELLYSA STERN CAHOY, children's librarian, Burlington Public Library, Burlington, Massachusetts

DEBORAH CHAMBERLAIN, research associate, Norwood, Massachusetts

DAVID S. CHAPIN, M.D., director of gynecology, Beth Israel Deaconness Medical Center, Boston, Massachusetts

DONALD J. COHEN, M.D., director, professor of psychiatry, pediatrics, and psychology, Yale University Child Study Center, New Haven, Connecticut

EILEEN COSTELLO, M.D., assistant clinical director of pediatrics, Boston University School of Medicine; pediatrician, Dorchester House, Dorchester, Massachusetts

SALLY CRISSMAN, science educator, Shady Hill School, Cambridge, Massachusetts

MARY DOMINGUEZ, science teacher, Shady Hill School, Cambridge, Massachusetts

KELLY DONNELL, assistant director, Teacher Training Course, Shady Hill School, Cambridge, Massachusetts

NANCY DROOKER, psychologist and sexuality education consultant, San Francisco, California

JENNIFER FRIEDMAN, teacher, Mather School, Boston, Massachusetts

NICKI NICHOLS GAMBLE, president, Planned Parenthood League of Massachusetts, Boston, Massachusetts

HILARY GRAND, elementary school teacher, New York, New York

BEN H. HARRIS, elementary school teacher, New York, New York

BILL HARRIS, parent, Cambridge, Massachusetts

DAVID B. HARRIS, elementary school teacher, New York, New York

GERALD HASS, M.D., pediatrician, Cambridge, Massachusetts, physician in chief, South End Community Health Center, Boston, Massachusetts

ROBYN HEILBRUN, parent, Salt Lake City, Utah

DORIS B. HELD, M.ED., psychotherapist, Harvard Medical School, member of the Governor's Commission on Gay and Lesbian Youth for the Commonwealth of Massachusetts, Cambridge, Massachusetts

PAT HORN, teacher, Shady Hill School, Cambridge, Massachusetts

MICHAEL ISKOWITZ, policy and strategy architect, Washington, D.C.

SUZAN KAITZ, chair, The PURPOSE Campaign, Planned Parenthood League of Massachusetts, Boston, Massachusetts

LESLIE M. KANTOR, M.P.H., vice president for education, Planned Parenthood of New York City, New York, New York

LARRY KESSLER, executive director, AIDS Action Committee of Massachusetts, Boston, Massachusetts

RONA KNIGHT, PH.D., child, adolescent, and adult analyst, Newton, Massachusetts

PHILIP KREMEN, barrister, London, England

ROBERT A. LEVINE PH.D., professor of education, human development, and anthropology, Harvard University Graduate School of Education, Cambridge, Massachusetts

ELIZABETH A. LEVY, children's book author, New York, New York

JAY LEVY, M.D., professor, department of medicine, research associate, Cancer Research Institute, University of California School of Medicine, San Francisco, California

JENIFER LORD, social worker, British Agencies for Adoption and Fostering, London, England

CAROL LYNCH, director of education and training, Planned Parenthood League of Massachusetts, Boston, Massachusetts

STEVEN MARANS, PH.D., assistant professor of psychoanalysis, Yale University Child Study Center, New Haven, Connecticut

WENDY DALTON MARANS, M.SC., associate research scientist, Yale University Child Study Center, New Haven, Connecticut

KIM MARSHALL, principal, Mather School, Boston, Massachusetts

LINDA C. MAYES, M.D., associate professor of child psychiatry/pediatrics and psychology, Yale University Child Study Center, New Haven, Connecticut

JENNIFER MCGUINN, teacher, Shady Hill School, Cambridge, Massachusetts

RONALD JAMES MOGLIA, ED.D., professor, Department of Health, New York University, New York, New York

PATRICIA C. MORRIS, teacher, Mather School, Boston, Massachusetts

ELI NEWBERGER, M.D., director, Family Development Program, Children's Hospital, Boston, Massachusetts

JUNE NICHOLS, R.N., Walpole, Massachusetts

JAN PARADISE, M.D., associate professor of pediatrics, Boston University School of Medicine, Boston, Massachusetts

DEB POLANSKY, teacher, Shady Hill School, Cambridge, Massachusetts

GALE PRYOR, author, Belmont, Massachusetts

JEFFREY PUDNEY, PH.D., research associate, Harvard Medical School, Boston, Massachusetts

LOUISE RICE R.N., director of education, AIDS Action Committee of Massachusetts, Boston, Massachusetts

LAURA RILEY, M.D., obstetrician/gynecologist, director, Ob/Gyn Infectious Diseases, Massachusetts General Hospital, Boston, Massachusetts

SUKEY ROSENBAUM, parent, New York, New York

HERMINE SARKISSIAN, pediatrician, Yerevan, Armenia

DEBORAH SCHOEBERLEIN, director, Redefining Actions & Decisions Educational Programs, Carbondale, Colorado

CAROL SEPKOSKI, PH.D., developmental psychologist, Cambridge, Massachusetts

DEIDRE SHEEDY, parent, Concord, Massachusetts

RACHEL SKVIRSKY, PH.D., associate professor of biology, University of Massachusetts, Boston, Massachusetts

CATHERINE STEINER-ADAIR, PH.D., psychologist, Lexington, Massachusetts

JULIE STEVENSON, teacher, The San Francisco School, San Francisco, California

TRISH MOYLAN TORRUELLA, M.P.H., sexuality education consultant, New York, New York

EDWARD Z. TRONICK, PH.D., chief, Child Development Unit, Children's Hospital, Boston, Massachusetts

BARRY ZUCKERMAN, M.D., chairman, Department of Pediatrics, Boston University School of Medicine, Boston City Hospital, Boston, Massachusetts

PAMELA MEYER ZUCKERMAN, M.D., pediatrician, Brookline, Massachusetts

Thanks to all our colleagues at Candlewick Press and Walker Books. And a very special thanks to **AMY EHRLICH, LIZ GAVRIL, JULIE BUSHWAY, ANNE MOORE, GILL WILLIS, WENDY BOASE,** and **RUTH WILLIAMS.**

R. H. H. and M. E.

INDEX

There are so-ooo many A-MAZING things in this book! And right here is a list of all those things, with their page numbers, so you can find out WHAT you want to find out.

One last thing. The **BOLD** numbers are the page numbers WHERE you can find out what a word or words mean!

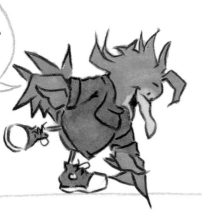

INDEX

Ii

identical. *See* identical twins; triplets; quadruplets; quintuplets
identical twins, **54–55**
incubator, **60**
infection(s), 39, 73. *See also* HIV; virus

Ll

labia, **15**
labour, **56–57**
lanugo, **44**
lesbian, 31–**32**, 65. *See also* gay; homosexual
love, 28, 29, **30–33**, 67, 68

Mm

making love, **29**, 31. *See also* sexual intercourse
male, **10**–11, 26–27, 31, 32, 44, 62. *See also* gender
marriage, 64
masturbation, **69**
menstruation, **19–21**
midwife, 56, 57, 58
milk. *See* breast milk; cow's milk; formula; soy milk
miscarriage, **42**

Nn

navel, **47, 58**. *See also* tummy-button
needle(s), 72, 73
nurse, 7, 53, 70, 73

Oo

ovary (ovaries), **11**, 12, **15**, 18, 20, 21, 34, 35, 39

Pp

pad, **21**
parent(s), 7, 29, 31, 58, 60, 62–63, 64–67, 68, 69. *See also* birth father; birth mother; birth parent(s); family; foster parent(s)
penis, 12, **17**, 23, 24, 25, 28, 34, 39
period. *See* menstruation
pill, **39**
placenta, **47**, 48, 49, 59
poo. *See* solid waste
prem. *See* premature baby
pregnancy, **40**–45, 46–49, 50–53, 73
pregnant, **40**. *See also* pregnancy
premature baby, **60**
private parts, **68**, 69, 70. *See also* body, female; body, male
prostate gland, **17**, 23
puberty, female, **11**, **12–13**, 14–15, 18, 20, 21
puberty, male, **11**, **12–13**, 16–17, 24, 25

Qq

quadruplets, 54, **55**
quintuplets, 54, **55**

Rr

reproduction, **8**

Ss

scrotum, **17**
semen, **23**, 24, 25, 34
seminal vesicles, **17**, 23
sex, **26–29**, 30. *See also* gender; having sex; making love; sexual intercourse
sexual abuse, **70–71**
sexual attraction, **32**
sexual intercourse, **28–29**, 34, 38, 39, 73
solid waste, 15, 17
soy milk, 61
sperm, **9**, 11, 12, 17, 19, 21, 22–25, 26, 28, 34–39, 54, 55, 62, 63, 66. *See also* cell(s)

Tt

stepparent(s), 65
stomach, 10, 14, 16, 41, 48, 51
straight, 31–**32**

Tt

tampon, **21**
testicles, **11**, 12, **17**, 22, 24, 25
triplets, 54, **55**
tummy-button, 14, 16, 41, **47**, 57, **58**
twins, 53, **54–55**, 63

Uu

ultrasound, **53**
umbilical cord, **47**, 48, 49, 58, 59
urethra, **15**, **17**, 20, 23, 25
urine, 15, 17, 20, 25, 49
uterus, **15**, 19, 20, 34–35, 37, 38, 40, 44, 56, 57, 59, 66

Vv

vagina, **15**, 19, 20, 21, 28, 34, 38, 57, 59
vas deferens, **17**, 22–23
vernix, **44**
virus, **72**. *See also* HIV; infection(s)
vulva, 12, **15**

Ww

wee. *See* urine
wet dream, **25**
womb, 40, **41**. *See also* uterus

Xx

X chromosome, **62**

Yy

Y chromosome, **62**

Zz

zygote, **37**

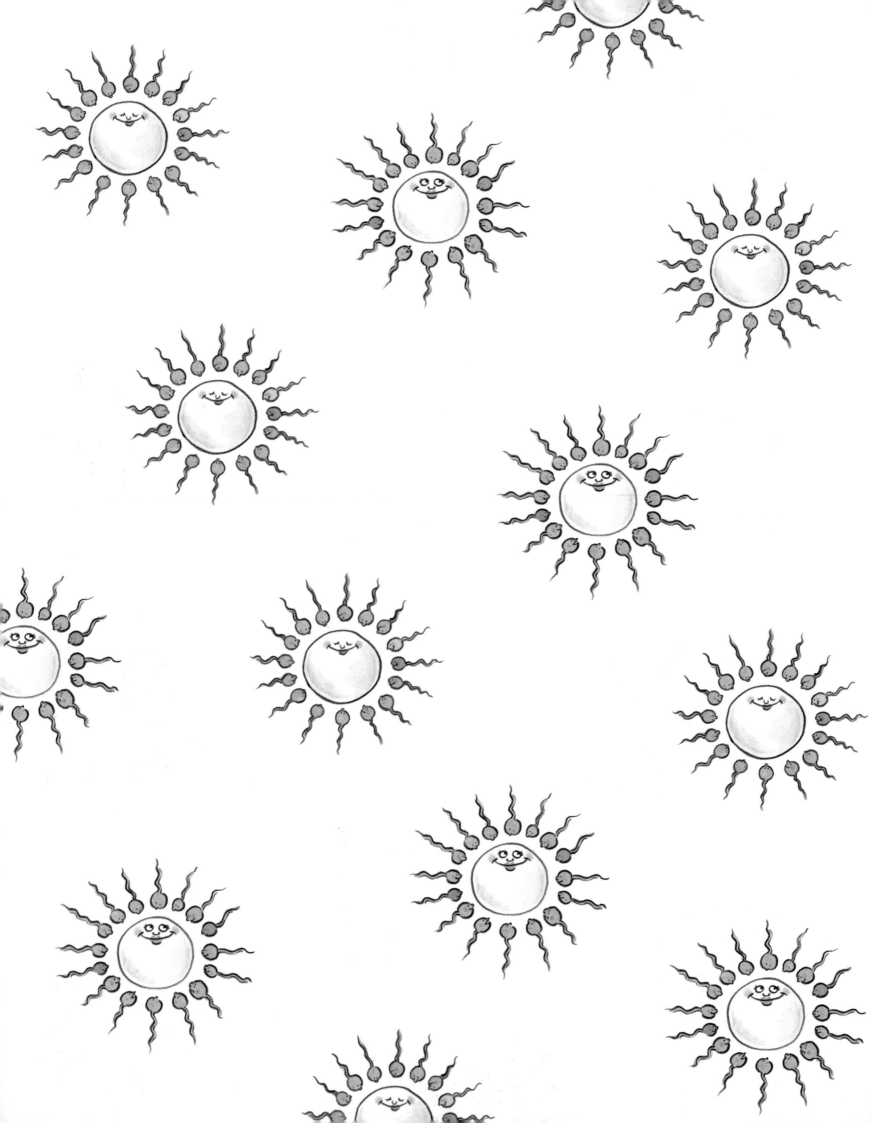

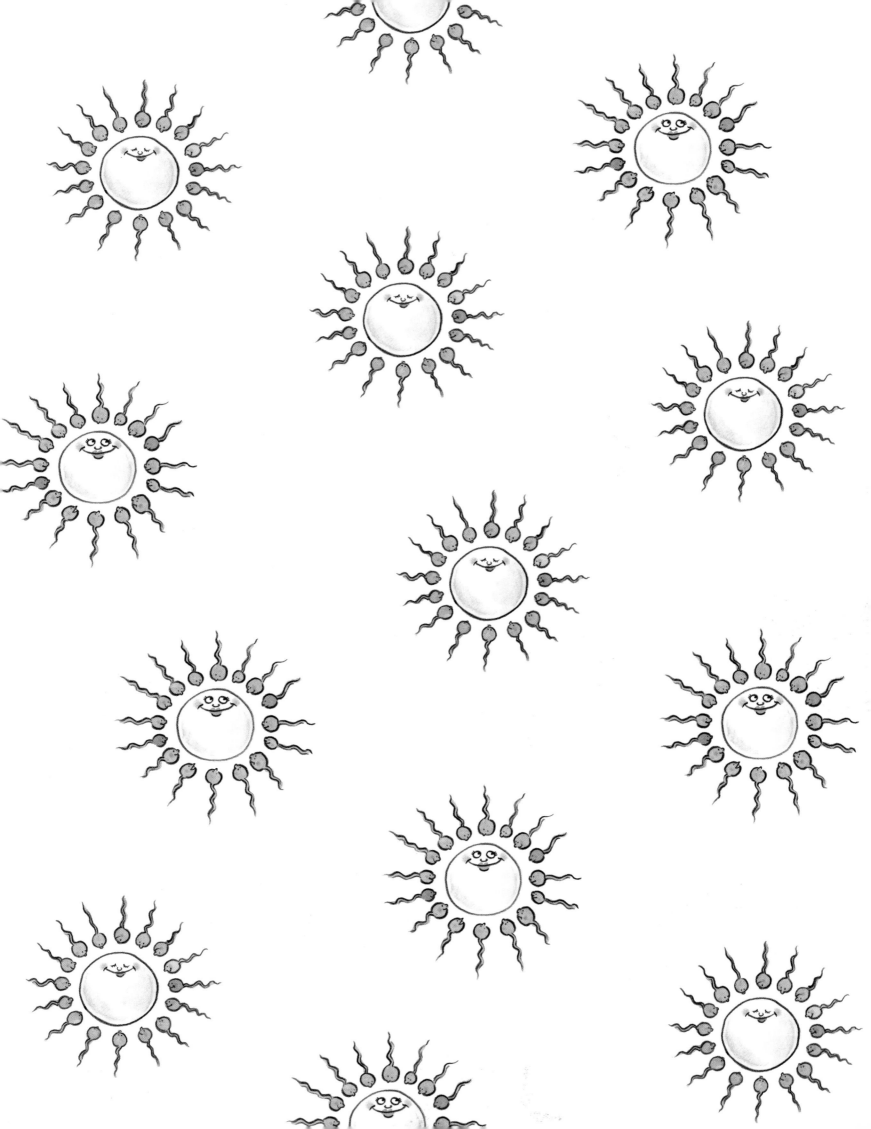

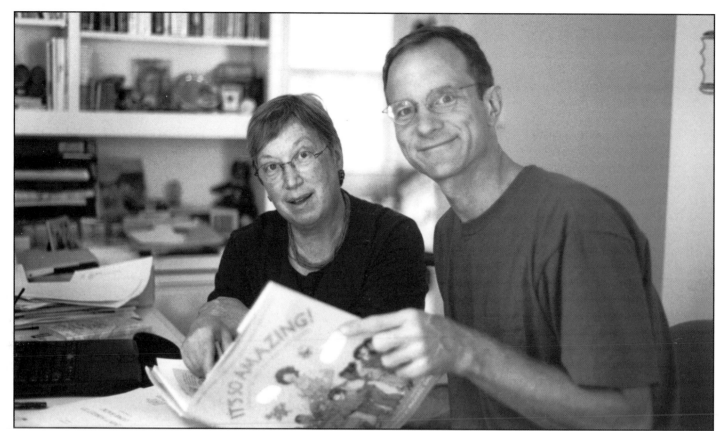

Robie H. Harris

began her career as a teacher at the Bank Street College of Education's School for Children. Her interest in child development issues and the experience of being a parent made her realize "how difficult but necessary it is to talk with children and teenagers about sex and answer questions about this complicated topic. I wanted my kids to stay healthy, so I had to give them accurate information." She says, "My challenge in writing *Let's Talk About Where Babies Come From* was to weave the fascinating and complicated science facts about reproduction and birth into the story of the egg and the sperm, and to communicate to children in an honest and simple way how amazing this story really is!" Robie H. Harris is the well-known author of *Happy Birth Day!*, *Hi New Baby!* and *Let's Talk About Sex* – all illustrated by Michael Emberley. She lives in Massachusetts, USA.

Michael Emberley,

son of children's book illustrator Ed Emberley, attended the Rhode Island School of Design. He is the illustrator of many books for children, including *Happy Birth Day!*, *Hi New Baby!* and *Let's Talk About Sex* – all written by Robie H. Harris. He says that while creating the illustrations for *Let's Talk About Where Babies Come From*, he "tried to delicately balance age-appropriateness, absolute accuracy, honesty and just plain fun." Michael Emberley lives in Massachusetts, USA.